Mindfulness and Eating Disorders across the Lifespan

This important and well researched volume examines the clinical phenomenon of eating disorders, exploring their longitudinal risk trajectory and introducing the Mindful Emotion Regulation – Approach (MER-A) as a starting point for intervention.

The book reviews various eating problems that can originate from the earliest perinatal phase to early adolescence, and through the MER-A framework focuses on how the principles of mindfulness and the related theoretical and clinical bases underlying the construct of emotional regulation can guide the clinician to a deeper understanding of a patient's disordered eating. Featuring reflections on clinical cases, it includes coverage of patients' difficulties in regulating emotions, their relationships with various eating behaviours and their associated interpersonal features.

Mindfulness and Eating Disorders across the Lifespan represents an attempt to provide a complete appreciation of this complex and multifaceted topic, making it of great importance to psychotherapists and related mental health professionals working with eating disorders.

Gaia de Campora has worked in the field of perinatal and developmental psychology for the past fifteen years, dedicating her expertise to research and clinical work with individuals and families. She is currently enrolled as Adjunct Professor at the University of Turin, where her teaching activities are mainly focused on the recognition of risk factors and the psychodiagnoses of perinatal disorders.

Giulio Cesare Zavattini is former Full Professor in Psychopathology of Couple Relationships at the Faculty of Medicine and Psychology, Sapienza, University of Rome. He is a Psychoanalyst of Società Psicoanalitica Italiana, the International Psychoanalytic Society, the Tavistock Institute of Medical Psychology and the International Association of Couple and Family Psychoanalysis. He has also written several books and essays on attachment, parental and romantic relationships.

Mindfulness and Eating Disorders across the Lifespan

Assessment and Intervention through the Emotion Regulation Paradigm

Edited by
Gaia de Campora and
Giulio Cesare Zavattini

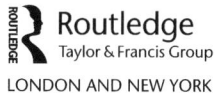

Routledge
Taylor & Francis Group

LONDON AND NEW YORK

First published 2021
by Routledge
2 Park Square, Milton Park, Abingdon, Oxon OX14 4RN

and by Routledge
605 Third Avenue, New York, NY 10158

Routledge is an imprint of the Taylor & Francis Group, an informa business

Translated by Leonardo De Pascalis.

Published in Italian by Società editrice il Mulino 2016 with the title *Mindfulness e disturbi alimentari* © by Società editrice il Mulino, Bologna 2016

British Library Cataloguing-in-Publication Data
A catalogue record for this book is available from the British Library

Library of Congress Cataloging-in-Publication Data
A catalog record has been requested for this book

ISBN: 978-0-367-72290-6 (hbk)
ISBN: 978-0-367-72289-0 (pbk)
ISBN: 978-1-003-15426-6 (ebk)

Typeset in Times New Roman
by Taylor & Francis Books

Contents

List of illustrations   viii
List of contributors   ix
Acknowledgements   xi
Foreword   xii

Introduction   1
GAIA DE CAMPORA AND GIULIO CESARE ZAVATTINI

PART I
Regulation and nutrition   3

1   From the prenatal phase to early adulthood: Risk factors and
    regulatory processes in the individual's lifespan   5
    GAIA DE CAMPORA AND GIULIO CESARE ZAVATTINI

    1. The meaning of nutrition 5
    2. The first nine months of life: foetal programming hypothesis 6
    3. Parental state of mind in relation to eating 7
    4. Regulatory processes in the cycle of life 8
    5. Conclusions 10

2   Mindful Emotion Regulation – Approach (MER-A):
    A theoretical model for the treatment of eating disorders
    during development   12
    GAIA DE CAMPORA

    1. Which treatment and which context? 12
    *2. Mindful Emotion Regulation – Approach (MER-A): reading
    model and intervention on the ED in children and
    adolescents 16*

3. Conclusions 17

PART II
Assessment and treatment across the life course 19

3 Overweight and obesity risk in the first three years of life 21
GAIA DE CAMPORA AND GIULIO CESARE ZAVATTINI

  1. Overweight – from the perinatal phase to the first three years of
  life: state of the art, research prospects, and prevention 21
  2. Prevention starts with the relationship: the use of video
  feedback at home 24
  3. Sara and Matteo: a story of "power" 26
  4. Conclusions 29

4 Infantile anorexia and Post-Traumatic Feeding Disorder in
early infancy 33
LOREDANA LUCARELLI

  1. Introduction 33
  2. Relevant clinical aspects of the avoidant/restrictive food intake
  disorder: Infantile Anorexia and Post-Traumatic Feeding
  Disorder 36
  3. Infantile Anorexia and Post-Traumatic Eating Disorder:
  parent–child interactions and clinical intervention 43

5 Food refusal in preschool-age children 52
ELENA TROMBINI AND GIANCARLO TROMBINI

  1. Problems with eating and emotion regulation in preschool
  age 52
  2. The psychotherapeutic intervention 54
  3. Focal Play-Therapy with children and their parents: theory and
  technique 55
  4. Focal Play-Therapy and narrative play 60
  5. "Getting in the game" with children and parents through Focal
  Play-Therapy: clinical vignettes 62
  6. Conclusive thoughts 67

6 Food selectivity and pre-adolescence 72
ANNA MARIA DELOGU

1. Pre-adolescence: a matter of boundaries 72
2. Food selectivity: brief nosographic notes 73
3. Family-based interventions 74
4. A clinical case 79
5. Conclusions 86

7   Bulimia and adolescence   90
    MOJGAN KHADEMI AND HEIDI MILLER BRUNETTO

1. Bulimia and adolescence: theoretical overview 90
2. The clinical approach 91
3. Case discussion 93
4. Conclusions 96

References   98
Index   117

Illustrations

Figures

5.1 Gigetto is looking at the delicious food he would like to eat: those
    little pieces, brought to the mouth at first, then slip in his tummy   57
5.2 Gigetto is feeling full and he would like to evacuate. Those little pieces
    of food become stools, and they are now ready to fall into the toilet   57
5.3 After Gigetto has eaten and evacuated, he is free to play, eat
    again, and go to sleep   58

Table

4.1 Eating disorders between 0 and 3 years of age (Axis I: DC:0–3R,
    Zero To Three 2005, 2008)   37

Contributors

Gaia de Campora has worked in the field of perinatal and developmental psychology for the past fifteen years, dedicating her expertise to research and clinical work with individuals and families. She is currently enrolled as Adjunct Professor at the University of Turin, where her teaching activities are mainly focused on the recognition of risk factors and the psycho-diagnoses of perinatal disorders.

Anna Maria Delogu (PhD) is a Psychologist and Psychotherapist. She mainly works with couples and families with particular attention to issues related to attachment and to an integrated clinical approach to psychopathology. Her research interests are especially dedicated to the attachment and reflective functioning underlying eating disorders in adolescence.

Mojgan Khademi (PsyD) is a Licensed Psychologist and Board-Certified Psychoanalyst and Fellow of the American Board of Psychoanalysis (FABP). She was the recipient of the American Psychoanalytic Association's Edith Sabshin Teaching Award in 2015, given in recognition of outstanding contributions as an educator. She has a private practice in San Diego and is co-chair of the Education Committee at the San Diego Psychoanalytic Center (SDPC), focused on post-doctorate education in psychoanalysis.

Loredana Lucarelli (PsyD) is Full Professor in Dynamic and Developmental Psychopathology and Director of the Department of Pedagogy, Psychological Sciences, Philosophy at University of Cagliari, IT. Her scientific activity concerns: diagnostic systems and childhood assessment, perinatality and transition to parenthood, relationships between infant attachment and parental psychopathology, developmental feeding and eating disorders.

Heidi Miller Brunetto (PsyD) is a Clinical Psychologist at Neighborhood Healthcare in San Diego, CA. She practices health psychology in an integrated primary care clinic. She has special interests in women's issues and has contributed in studies focused on deficit in mentalisation as risk factors for eating disorders.

Elena Trombini (PsyD) is Full Professor in Dynamic Psychology and Vice Dean for Students, Department of Psychology, University of Bologna. She is the founding director of the Psychological Consultation Centre for Children and Parents and of the Research Laboratory 'Dina Vallino' (Department of Psychology, University of Bologna). Psychologist and psychodynamic psychotherapist, her primary research and clinical interests are the prevention and treatment of eating disorders in both children and adults.

Giancarlo Trombini (MD, PsyD) is Emeritus in Clinical Psychology, University of Bologna. He spent over fifty years dedicating his research and clinical interests to the integration of a medical and psychological point of view. He has been the author of over 300 scientific publications, and is an active member of the Italian Psychoanalytic Society (SPI) and the International Psychoanalytic Association (IPA).

Giulio Cesare Zavattini is former Full Professor in Psychopathology of Couple Relationships at the Faculty of Medicine and Psychology, Sapienza, University of Rome. He is a Psychoanalyst of Società Psicoanalitica Italiana, the International Psychoanalytic Society, the Tavistock Institute of Medical Psychology and the International Association of Couple and Family Psychoanalysis. He has also written several books and essays on attachment, parental and romantic relationships.

Acknowledgements

We are deeply grateful to Leonardo De Pascalis (PhD), Lecturer in Developmental Psychopathology at the Department of Psychological Science, University of Liverpool, for his outstanding care and help in translating our book.

Foreword

How many names are given to what we refer to as eating disorders, to obey the irresistible need to name, classify, divide (taxonomy) and then reconnect (nosology) phenomena observed and considered to be pathological?

According to the diagnostic classification of mental health and developmental disorders of infancy and early childhood, at least six clinical conditions can be identified for the age group ranging from birth to three years (Zero to Three 2005):

- feeding disorder of state regulation (homeostasis)
- feeding disorder of caregiver–infant reciprocity
- infantile anorexia
- sensory food aversions
- feeding disorder associated with concurrent medical condition
- post-traumatic feeding disorder

For the paediatric age, up to the beginning of adolescence, at least eight diagnostic categories are described (Lask & Bryant-Waugh 2013; Nicholls & Bryant-Waugh 2009):

- food refusal and pervasive refusal syndrome
- selective eating
- food avoidance emotional disorder
- food phobias
- functional dysphagia
- early onset anorexia nervosa
- early onset bulimia nervosa
- early onset binge eating disorder

The DSM-5, aimed primarily at adolescence and adulthood, also lists eight types of feeding and eating disorders (American Psychiatric Association 2013):

- pica
- rumination disorder

- avoidant-restrictive food intake disorder
- anorexia nervosa
- bulimia nervosa
- binge eating disorder
- other specified feeding or eating disorder
- unspecified feeding or eating disorder

The eleventh revision of the International Classification of Diseases (ICD-11), in relation to eating disorders, has followed the DSM-5 with some differences (Forney et al. 2016; Thiels & Deb 2014).

Finally, to the more or less widely accepted official classifications, one should add the continuous suggestions for new diagnostic categories such as orthorexia nervosa, night eating syndrome, emetophobia, purging disorder, etc.

The book, edited by Gaia de Campora and Giulio Cesare Zavattini, is not structured according to a diagnostic criterion but many of the names mentioned above appear frequently throughout its seven chapters. As a text, it is above all aimed towards the treatment and prevention of eating disorders in childhood and adolescence and, therefore, considers the various clinical conditions according to a shared and trans-diagnostic perspective.

Furthermore – and rightly so – much space is dedicated by the authors to obesity, a condition as important as it is still poorly defined (Bosello & Cuzzolaro 2013; Bosello, Donataccio, & Cuzzolaro 2016). Some recent epidemiological findings concerning obesity offer useful background elements to understand the relevance of this volume and to introduce its reading.

Through the method of pooled analysis, a study published in 2016 in the *Lancet* journal examined the change in adult human body weight between 1975 and 2014 (Collaboration NCDRF 2016). Data from 1698 population studies on more than 19 million people from 200 different nations were used. Just a few findings are enough to clearly illustrate the great change that took place over the course of forty years: the global average body mass index (BMI $-$ kg/m2) rose from 21.7 to 24.2 in men and from 22.1 to 24.4 in women, while the overall prevalence of obesity (BMI >30) increased from 3.2% to 10.8% in men and from 6.4% to 14.9% in women and, if the current trends persist, by 2025 the global prevalence of obesity will be 18% in men and 21% in women. Approximately one fifth of the world adult population will be affected by obesity. During the same period of time (1975–2014), the global prevalence of malnutrition instead decreased from 13.8% to 8.8% in men and from 14.6% to 9.7% in women. Thus, the world has gone from a time when severely malnourished people were twice as many as those suffering from obesity to one in which, for the first time in the history of the Homo Sapiens species, the number of obese people exceeds that of malnourished ones.

Together with these changes in weight and adiposity, many people live longer than in the past: the average life expectancy, calculated globally, has increased from less than 59 years in 1975 to over 71, forty years later.

However, speaking of the latter increase, not all the added years are of good quality. HALE (Healthy Life Expectancy) is a valuable statistical indicator that measures how morbidity (getting sick from diseases that leave sequelae and permanent disabilities) changes with respect to mortality trends. It is used in epidemiology to evaluate and compare public health problems in different countries and/or different historical periods.

In another large study, Joshua Salomon and colleagues calculated HALE in 187 different countries and its change from 1990 to 2010 (Salomon et al. 2012). They found that healthy life expectancy increased but far less than overall life expectancy. In other words, life expectancy increased substantially, but much less progress was made in reducing the burden of long-lasting sequelae and disabilities due to non-fatal illnesses.

Commenting on these general indicators, George Davey Smith concluded that, in the decades around the turn of the millennium, the population of this world has become overall fatter, lives longer but many years are compromised by chronic diseases and disabilities. Furthermore, social inequalities in terms of economic well-being have increased dramatically (Smith et al., 2016). All this has important and easily understandable consequences on health policy decisions and their economic repercussions.

Regarding eating disorders and obesity as well, treatments in the last half century have brought about a reduction in mortality but had a smaller impact on permanent sequelae and on long-term disabilities (Cuzzolaro 2014; Steinhausen 2009). The study of effective, early and economically sustainable interventions for the prevention and treatment of eating and weight disorders – the subject of this volume – appears increasingly necessary.

The explosion of obesity has been progressive, pandemic and so far unstoppable. Looking at developmental trends, the prevalence of childhood obesity has doubled over the past thirty years and adolescent obesity has even quadrupled in both the United States and various other countries.

It should be emphasised that overweight in childhood and adolescence is an important risk factor not only for obesity in adulthood, and for the many obesity-related diseases, but also for the development of depressive symptoms, of a negative body image, of serious eating disorders and of dangerous weight control practices (self-induced vomiting, abuse of laxatives and drugs, excessive physical exercise, etc.) (Lebow, Sim, & Kransdorf 2015).

In the same short period of time during which, due to excessive food offers and a sedentary lifestyle, the world has become increasingly obesogenic (Watson et al. 2016), there has also been a general complication of the relationship human beings have with food and abnormal eating behaviours, harmful to physical and mental health, have spread throughout all seasons of life and especially among the youngest.

In children and adolescents, nutrition and growth are connected through the obvious, direct and quantitative relationship between caloric intake, weight and body composition. But, as this book correctly reminds us, the biological mechanisms of homeostatic regulation of the energy balance are modulated and possibly altered by various factors, starting as early as during the prenatal period. Gradually, at a conscious and unconscious level, the following come into play: the lifestyle of parents, family interactions, the peer groups, the socio-economic context, the cultural background, the more or less effective development of the ability to control and manage emotions and impulses, the mental body image with its load of insecurities and distress. And the relationship of the young human with nourishment and the caregiver very quickly becomes the privileged theatre of intra- and inter-personal conflicts.

An extensive scientific literature has dealt with and continues to address the problem of the treatment and prevention of eating and body weight disorders, which are deeply linked to each other (Haines et al. 2010; Wilksch et al. 2015). The book edited by Gaia de Campora and Giulio Cesare Zavattini enters this scientific domain with originality and richness of content. It explores a territory of research and therapeutic applications developed in recent years and illustrates them through clinical cases. A few examples:

- interventions centred on strengthening the ability to pay attention to the here and now, to the present moment (mindfulness-based), such as focal play-therapy with children and parents, a technique belonging to the methodology of mindful approaches for emotion regulation.
- the use of video recordings (video-feedback), within a parent–child psychotherapy, with the aim of preventing the onset of overweight in children, counteracting the intergenerational transmission of obesity and treating problematic eating behaviours as early as during the perinatal period and in early infancy.
- mentalisation-based family therapy in pre-adolescence.

This last concept deserves a brief historical reflection, as it has also become an important bridging construct, shared by psychoanalysis and cognitive psychology, by ethology and neuroscience. It is a common thread of this book that also returns in the seventh and last chapter, dedicated to the integrated psychodynamic approach in the treatment of adolescent bulimia nervosa. A treatment approach that is integrated in the sense that it attempts to insert cognitive–behavioural techniques into a model of psychoanalytic derivation.

But when did we start talking about mentalisation? And in what sense?

The term mentalisation was introduced by the Swiss psychologist Édouard Claparède in the first decades of the twentieth century to indicate the ability to become aware, recognise and process conflicting emotions and tensions (Claparède 1930). Claparède's original words still sound clear: "This way of seeing allows us to understand the usefulness of the mentalisation of feelings ... If feelings are a mentalised process, this enables them to also become the object of reflection, of comparison" (p. 6). Around the mid-twentieth century, Wilfred Ruprecht Bion spoke of the alpha function of the psychic apparatus to indicate an analogous concept, the way in which the psyche creates symbols to represent emotional states and elaborates them (Bion 1963). The alpha function is the mental activity that, starting from the beta elements (sensory, proto-emotional inputs) weaves thought, first as mental images (pictograms), then as cognitive operations and words (alpha elements). According to this vision, failures in Bion's alphabetisation (which is not so far from Claparède's mentalisation) open the door to psychotic breaks, somatisations, episodes of acting out without thought. In the second half of the last century, the Parisian psychosomatic school used the concept of operational thought (Marty, De M'Uzan, & David 1963) to indicate a stable defect in the capacity for mentalisation (Marty 1991), that is, in the capacity to recognise, distinguish, elaborate and communicate through language one's own emotional states and those observed in others, for example in a child. In the 1970s, Peter Sifneos used the term alexithymia to refer to the same defect (Sifneos 1973). According to this theory, the capacity for mentalisation is:

a Impaired in people with serious alexithymic traits, who tend to discharge emotional tensions through other channels, e.g., somatically.
b Physiologically insufficient during development and, especially, in infancy, when the vicarious function belongs to the adult, in the psycho-somatic caregiver–infant dyad (Kreisler, Fain, & Soulé 1974).

And what if the adult fails the task? It is then that the various treatments try to intervene. I would like to add, with the humility recommended by Bion: to wait for a pattern to emerge, to be able not to know in order to allow it.

Massimo Cuzzolaro
Formerly at Sapienza University of Rome, Italy
Editor-in-chief, *Eating and Weight Disorders –
Studies on Anorexia Bulimia Obesity*

Introduction

Gaia de Campora and Giulio Cesare Zavattini

The ability of favouring some foods over others, together with the eating behaviour associated with them, begin to emerge at conception and continue to develop throughout the whole cycle of an individual's life. The development of this individual characteristic implies a complex interchange between biological and environmental factors. Many studies have demonstrated that there are children who are hard-wired towards "beneficial" nutrients, for example sweet foods that represent access to calories and therefore hint at an idea of availability of resources necessary for survival, or rather attracted towards bitter foods, which according to an ontogenetic approach, represent a potential danger, as in the case of poisons.

Next to a theory that stresses the idea of precocious "programming", there is a tradition that focuses on the progressive development of these characteristics and that sees the emerging of post-natal preferences connected to taste, smell, and texture inside the uterus, in the beginning of the relation between mother and child. The child has the defined ability to discern among the different sensorial characteristics of food from the last weeks of gestational life, in fact many food habits apparent in the first days of perinatal life are valid and reliable indicators of food habits in adult life.

Obviously, many transitions happen between one phase and another in the life cycle; that is the case, for example, of the food phobia that occurs in babies during the weaning period, when passing from milk to solid foods, a phase in which the affective components are indistinguishable from dietary ones. In fact, the behaviour of strong refusal observed in this phase has a crucial adaptive function, aiming at preventing the separation from the parent and guaranteeing instead the continuity of a *safe* and *familiar* food environment that guarantees the parent's closeness, removing the risk of "experimenting" with potentially harmful new foods. The acceptance of change, in fact, similarly to the preference for flavours that babies are exposed to during pregnancy, inevitably passes through the inter- and extra-uterine environment, and therefore, through the relationship with the outside, a communication that occurs from the very beginning through the attachment bond with the caregiver. In fact, the parent, by building a relation with her own child, introduces the baby to the adoption of a new language – the language of food – in relation to which the affective exchange builds the foundation for the child's future abilities in regulating their own physical (hunger or satiety) and emotional states.

The proposal of our book focuses on the meeting point of the various elements known to us today, on the consideration that transitional issues and real food disorders have an early history, almost an "ancient" one, that goes back to the bond between parent and child during pregnancy, and which accompanies the individual throughout her life cycle.

More specifically, the model of intervention that we present here, the *Mindful Emotion Regulation – Approach* (MER-A) refers to the integration of two perspectives, *mindfulness* and *emotional regulation*, which focus on a few aspects that we deem very important in matters of food disorders and that we can summarize in the expression of "non-judgmental acceptance of the present moment, in light of the competences and of the individual difficulties in regulating our emotions and our relationship with food." We will see further on what we mean by this and how this expression can be reflected in the interventions applied in the area of food disorders.

In the following chapters, we will describe different food disorders and the distinctive defining phases of the life cycle, beginning with a first case dealing with a perinatal food disorder and concluding in the last chapter with a case of a food disorder in a teenager. The common thread of this volume is the focus on the processes of emotional regulation in order to promote and at the same time shift the reflection onto the present moment, on the here and now of eating behaviour.

Part I

Regulation and nutrition

From the prenatal phase to early adulthood

Risk factors and regulatory processes in the individual's lifespan

Gaia de Campora and Giulio Cesare Zavattini

1. The meaning of nutrition

The acts of feeding and eating are gestures that contain an incredible amount of information and meaning. In fact, eating behaviour is a sophisticated sensory-motor process which, since the early stages of life, changes and evolves throughout time, shifting from the necessity of being *together* with a meaningful other, usually a parent on whom we depend, to complete *autonomy* in food collection and intake. The line that virtually connects these two extremes, dependence and autonomy, covers a person's lifetime, and it characterizes the individual because of the constant presence of two interconnected elements that cannot be separated: the nutritional and the affective components. Because food is necessary to guarantee the survival of the child, strongly affective attitudes and behaviours are activated, especially when problems occur, for example, with food rejection. On the other hand, if during meals, both parent and child are engaged in together building the moment of food exchange, this *space* will become pleasant and the affective component will encourage the child to experiment with different kinds of food and different flavours.

The child's mind starts its development in the relationship with the caregiver during the feeding process (Candelori & Trumello 2015). A long tradition within dynamic psychology has dealt with the meaning of this feeding relationship in the evolution of mental well-being since the first days of life. We find an example of this in Bion's historical metaphor (1962), which symbolically compares the mental mechanisms of introjection/projection to the activities of the digestive systems, assimilation/evacuation. Accordingly, the state of discomfort and tension generated by the perception of hunger leads the child to experience a transient state of anguish, brought about by the child's inability to find a solution to their problem, which then leads them to tears (Quagliata 2002). This signal activates a response from the parent that aims at alleviating this painful state, bringing the child back to a condition of homeostasis, and simultaneously leaving an important trace in their mind: thanks to the maternal intervention, the state of anguish was accepted and digested, giving it a new, more tolerable meaning that is now part of the child's experience. According to the traditional approach of developmental psychology, these mechanisms of mental functioning represent the first attempts at building, together with the other person, the meaning of one's own experiences, a condition which later allows the child to separate from the caregiver, thanks to the newly acquired competencies/autonomies.

The first mental and emotional experiences are therefore strongly entangled with the nutritional ones, and together they constitute the basis for the individual's future eating habits.

2. The first nine months of life: foetal programming hypothesis

An essential contribution to the most recent scientific research consists of the observation of those factors that, at a very early stage, influence certain individual habits and behaviours, including eating habits. A considerable amount of evidence has been collected, and will be discussed in the following chapters, regarding the effects of early feeding interactions between mother and child, in defining risk or normative trajectories, following first infancy. What we define as Mother–Child early feeding interactions are those exchanges that help establish a nutritional rhythm in the infant since right after birth, whether the child is breastfed or given formula. An important part of this scientific discovery manifests itself in the re-definition of the word "early". In 1995, Barker proposed the *foetal programming hypothesis*, also known as Barker's hypothesis, which describes the existence of a sensitive period for foetal growth, which is supposed to characterize the early stages of pregnancy. In this early phase, structural and functional changes are caused by environmental stimuli. This aspect of the theory goes hand in hand with the epigenetic perspective, according to which our genes can express different ranges of physiological or morphological states in response to the environmental conditions. If the mother follows an inadequate diet while pregnant, this leads her infant towards systematically and severely impoverished long-term living conditions. The radical innovation of this scientific hypothesis is this: the conditions inside the womb do not simply represent risk factors for foetal health, but they are actual precursors of problems that will accompany the baby's existence, placing the child at a higher risk of diseases later in adulthood.

The type of nutrition received by the foetus triggers metabolic and developmental changes that are necessary for the foetus to adapt to the quality of life inside the uterus. Therefore, a scarce supply of nutrients and calories produces long-term changes as a result of restricted growth. Similarly, when one goes from a condition of malnutrition to one of overeating, this exposes the baby to future risks, such as diabetes and obesity, which are visible in the very early stages. Fast foetal growth increases the need of nutrients. This is not yet easily observable during pregnancy, but the effects are clearly evident after birth. Barker maintains that an excessive supply of nutrients during pregnancy leads to a loss of lean body mass that is linked to the production of amino acids, which from within the placenta, in turn, promote the ejection of maternal milk.

It is no coincidence that obese women have a harder time breastfeeding, and this is not just a consequence of a C-section, but it is an expression of a subtle regulatory mechanism between mother and children, where the latter are called, from early on, to push the environment towards their needs.

The results of this hypothesis do not stop here. There are in fact inter-generational effects connected to the nutrition and the weight of the indivi-dual, which link the mother's weight to the weight at birth of her children and grand-children. People have always been able to observe this relationship, but for the first time these effects are linked to environmental factors and not only to genetic heritage. This is why we chose an interdisciplinary approach as the only way to deeply understand the roots of eating problems.

3. Parental state of mind in relation to eating

If the mother's choice of food quality and quantity is so important for the baby's health from pregnancy to adult life, why are parents adopting unheal-thy nutritional habits?

As is documented by multiple studies, emotional and psychological states lead people to modify and/or intensify their nutritional habits, and we now call this mechanism *emotional eating*. Several studies have confirmed the connection between anxiety and depression and compulsive eating rather than complete withdrawal from food, but until recently, little attention has been paid to the specific phase of pregnancy. Generally, scientists think that gesta-tion functions as a trigger in the cases of women who show a history of eating disorders: they usually show improvement during pregnancy, but they revert to the same problems after giving birth. According to some, this improvement is due to the fact that pregnant women know that they are taking care of another being and they adopt a more caregiving behaviour. These data cannot be generalized and extended to the far more numerous subclinical population, which shows problems in this area without getting the clinician's attention. One example appears in the studies conducted by Wildes et al. (2008), where physical and emotional neglect in infants results in inadequate eating habits. In addition to this dysfunctional pattern, a series of related risks emerged, such as symptoms of depression, low self-esteem and substance abuse. These symptoms formed a non-specific condition in relation to the onset of psychopathology, regarding which the Authors note that interven-tions conducted at an early age produced significantly different and more favourable outcomes in adulthood for those individuals who accessed some form of intervention. The coexistence of comorbid symptoms that is found in cases of neglect and often poorly treated, seems to appear more frequently in cases of ill-treatment and abuse, affecting multiple systems in a cross-functional way: affective, behavioural, somatic, dissociative, and relational (Zucker, Spinazzola, Blaustein, & van der Kolk 2006). The study by Ringer and Crittenden (2007) highlighted how a third of their sample subjects, who mainly suffered from food disorders, reported unresolved traumatic events in early childhood, and seemed to point to a direct connection between the mental states of their mothers and their condition. In particular, it was clear that a trauma or an abuse that did not find a resolution in the parental function led to the formation of a symptom that was the direct expression of the inability to distinguish between emotional and physical needs, a competence that directly derives from the caregiver's inability to recognize and respond to the child's signals.

Notably, the mother's state of mind was characterized by a distancing attitude towards the attachment bond, which revealed itself in the tendency not to talk about the trauma or the abuse, as a strategy to protect the child from the impact of the event. In other words, the disguise of reality gave the illusion that the suffering created by those experiences could simply disappear; however, this approach caused instead the creation of a psychopathological nucleus that in the eating disorder symptoms found direct expression of the difficulties experienced by the child both individually and in the dyadic relationship.

The question at the beginning of this section seems to find some answers. A first hypothesis is that a certain attitude toward food is the answer to early childhood problems that never found a path toward resolution.

This explanation allows us to read these dynamics according to two different perspectives: (a) on the one hand, we can assume that eating problems are means of communication used by the child to signal an individual discomfort, and this, in time, will characterize his or her adult eating habits; (b) on the other hand, we can assume that food is the element through which traumas and/or mourning are transmitted from one generation to the next, allowing the passing on of the negative effects, from mother to child, and transforming food disorders into relational dysfunctions that permeate the individual's lifespan.

4. Regulatory processes in the cycle of life

In light of these observations, the hypothesis of intergenerational transmission proceeds on two parallel lines and is based on the empirical evidence from research in prenatal and perinatal medicine and in developmental psychopathology. This creates a *circular* motion that activates emotional and neurobiological processes that are intrinsically connected. In the study by Jahnke and Warschburger (2008), and later in the research conducted by Sleddens, Kremers, De Vries, and Thijs (2010), it emerged that emotional eating in one parent is associated with the child's request for food because of emotional needs, underlining the double role of genetic and behavioural mechanisms.

The early acquisition of this behaviour causes an alteration in the perception of our internal signals of hunger and satiety, reinforcing the sensibility toward external factors – like availability of food and/or presence of other people – which become regulatory elements of the beginning and of the end of a meal, as supported by Tan and Holub (2011).

The developmental cycle the individual embarks upon from birth in relation to eating habits relies on the constant alternation between internal and external contexts, where other elements, such as temperament, also contribute to etiopathogenesis. Throughout time, the child faces different adaptive competences, which include the progressive transition from a state of homeostasis, which mostly deals with physiological needs, to the building of the attachment with the caregiver, up until the separation and individuation from the caregiver toward individual autonomy.

This constant interweaving of innate and learned competences develops from the tactile, visual, auditory, and proprioceptive perceptions that characterize the relation between mother and child. In the beginning, the caregiver acts to restore in the child a state of calmness, which over time extends beyond the physiological dimension to affective and social relations. Synchrony, reciprocity, and harmony in the exchanges of food are the relational parameters according to which we must evaluate harmonic development or face the presence of pathology. The interactions between parent and child are dynamic processes that are constantly reworking each other. These interactions require a flexible evaluation that takes into account possible mismatches in the relationship, and they become of central importance depending on whether or not repair of the relationship follows (Busato Barbaglio & Mondello 2011).

This *constant alternating of mismatch and reparation processes* is at the foundation of self-regulation and interactive regulation, and is at the basis of the formation of eating habits. As Lichtenberg wrote, the internal perception of hunger that the child experiences requires an external empathic confirmation that validates and makes sense of the existence of this state, becoming part of the child's episodic and procedural memory and defining the event in his or her mind (Cuzzolaro, Piccolo & Speranza 2009).

Self-regulation and reciprocal regulation continue in a coordinated and alternating manner and, if this balance is maintained, the distinction between hunger (physiological state) and distress (emotional state) will be maintained. The development of the rhythm and of the ability to regulate one's appetite evolves because of the child's gradual achievements – like vocalizations and gaze direction – and because of the affective communication between the child and caregiver. In the early stages of life, child difficulties in communicating his or her own needs, or parental struggles in understanding and encouraging subsequent developmental stages may lead – among the other risk factors previously described – to the emergence of eating problems, of various degrees of severity, and their treatment can vary according to the theoretical model that is used to understand their roots.

5. Conclusions

The processes of self- and hetero-regulation represent multifaceted control systems and cover a role of primary importance in the different aspects of the life of the individual since birth (Graziano, Calkins, & Keane 2010). Many studies have shown the presence of a significant correlation among the regulatory processes that control individual abilities, and attentive abilities, sensitivity to control processes, and reward stimuli. These empirical observations have demonstrated how the individual's abilities to self-regulate take shape in time, becoming more integrated and sophisticated because of the developmental ability to monitor one's affective states and the tendency to enact the behaviours these states elicit.

The vast empirical evidence on the link between this construct and the individual's main developmental trajectories shows that, in addition to highlighting the predictive power of one aspect over the other, they point out the partial superimposition of these variables. Therefore, we can assume that the development of eating habits, together with the way we recognize and manage our emotional responses, are processes that accompany the individual throughout his/her lifespan, determining trajectories of risk or health that start at pregnancy. In this way, we can observe their reciprocal and constant influence, and finally, we can raise the question about the processes of linear causality and the meaning of their investigation, considering their circular patterns of operation.

Highlights

- Eating behaviour is a sophisticated sensory-motor process which changes and evolves throughout time, shifting from the necessity of being *together* with a meaningful other to complete *autonomy* in food collection and intake.
- Parent and child interactions require a flexible evaluation that takes into account possible mismatches in the relationship, and they become of central importance depending on whether or not repair of the relationship follows.
- The development of eating habits, together with the way we recognize and manage our emotional responses, are processes that accompany the individual throughout his/her lifespan, determining trajectories of risk or health that start at pregnancy.
- The *foetal programming hypothesis* describes the existence of a sensitive period for foetal growth, which is supposed to characterize the early stages of pregnancy: the conditions inside the womb do not simply

represent risk factors for foetal health, but they are actual precursors of problems that will accompany the baby's existence.

- There are intergenerational effects connected to the nutrition and weight of the individual, and for the first time these effects are linked to environmental factors and not just to genetic heritage.

Chapter 2

Mindful Emotion Regulation – Approach (MER-A)

A theoretical model for the treatment of eating disorders during development

Gaia de Campora

1. Which treatment and which context?

The late diagnosis and treatment of food disorders during development represents a serious risk for the health of children and adolescents, leading to a lower quality of life and imposing high prices to pay in their adulthood (Milnes, Piazza, & Carroll 2013; Williams, Riegel, Gibbons, & Field 2007). The persistence of eating disorders and the lack of early intervention almost inevitably lead to a worsening of the symptoms, with a considerable impact on the emotional, cognitive, and social development, and in general on the ability of the immune system to respond effectively (Lukens & Silverman 2014; Manikam & Perman 2000). Because of the multiplicity of factors involved in the etiopathogenesis of these disorders, *a biopsychosocial approach* should be considered, with the active involvement of different professionals, such as psychologists, medical doctors, nutritionists, and speech therapists.

Nowadays, there are different possible intervention strategies and, in particular, there are different factors upon which these strategies focus. Therefore, when considering the use of *evidence-based* interventions, it is necessary to keep in mind both the intrapersonal characteristics of the patient and the interpersonal ones, tied to family relationships, as essential elements to observe to obtain more effective long-term results.

Food disorders are characterized by different constellations of symptoms, and their onset can be the result of a multitude of personal histories. In the following chapters, diagnostic distinctions will be presented in detail, segmented mainly by the age in which the symptoms emerge. Because of this heterogeneous clinical manifestation, a clinical approach would need to cover different possibilities, adjusting itself to the specificity of the person, the family, and the disorder. Among the many alternatives, there are treatments that focus on changing eating behaviours, and therefore target elements such as the variety of accepted food and flavours, the reduction of specific behavioural problems, the improvement of meal organization and routines (Clawson & Elliott 2014). One example comes from the techniques derived from *Applied Behaviour Analysis* (ABA), which are used to manipulate and modify both the antecedents and the consequences of eating. Not all available techniques, however, even if clinically valid, have empirical evidence backing them up, and, most of all, not all approaches are accessible to families.

In a recent literature review about interventions in cases of paediatric eating disorders, it was shown that the treatment offered in hospitals to treat selective eating was inefficient (Lukens & Silverman 2014). Therefore, to treat *Avoidant/Restrictive Food Intake Disorders* (ARFIDs), which are the most common eating problem in children and which will be discussed in greater detail in the following chapters, it is necessary to resort to more effective interventions with regard to outcome and accessibility, both in terms of cost and duration. With this in mind, some researchers have applied already existing and scientifically validated approaches to the treatment of ARFIDs. For example, Fischer, Luiselli, and Dove (2015) described an intervention that integrated behavioural therapies and cognitive techniques. This method aimed at increasing feeding demands and at reinforcing food consumption, using relaxation techniques, guided visualizations, cognitive restructuring, as well as trying to increase the exploration of new foods, and reducing the levels of anxiety associated with them.

The problems surrounding this type of approach *are related to the age when the symptoms appear*. In fact, compared to adults and adolescents, infants show less motivation towards symptom reduction and are less able to adjust to and benefit from cognitive techniques. For these young patients, the clinical approach of choice should include techniques based on the principles of learning theory, as is the case for treating other behavioural disorders, such as disruptive behaviours, anxiety, and sleep disorders. These approaches are aimed at reinforcing positive elements by increasing their frequency and by decreasing the frequency of those behaviours that lead to rejection and avoidance, which, following these lines, gradually disappear.

As with any other childhood disorder, parents' reactions to their children's eating behaviours play a primary role in influencing their future behaviours. Low attunement in parental responses, including, for example, poor structuring of meal times, or providing food that is not age-appropriate (e.g., too liquid), or offering the child's favourite foods as a means to avoid food rejection, serve to reinforce the problems manifested by the child (Mitchell, Farrow, Haycraft, & Meyer 2013). This fact explains why, during hospitalization or day-hospital visits, these settings provide an opportunity for greater parental involvement, offering them the responsibility for the outcome of the treatment. Because social and environmental factors contribute to the persistence of behaviours specific to eating disorders, those techniques that focus on parental involvement can be particularly effective in hospitals, where the novelty of the environment can help break dysfunctional habits that are associated with being at home (Linsheid 2006).

In addition to the instructions that can be given to parents about how to propose meals, and which behaviours they should focus on – the so-called antecedents – the success of the intervention often depends on giving parents feedback about their behaviour during feeding interactions with their child, focusing attention on those elements that follow the meal. This approach has been studied in different settings and according to different perspectives, some of which will be later described in greater detail, and the results would seem to suggest its effectiveness (Anderson & McMillan 2001; McCartney, Anderson, English, & Horner 2005; Najdowski, Wallace, Doney, & Ghezzi 2003; Najdowski et al. 2010; Pizzo, Williams, Paul, & Riegel 2009; Seiverling, Williams, Sturmey, & Hart 2012; Sharp, Burrell, Jaquess 2014; Stark, Powers, Jelalian, Rape, & Miller 1994; Tarbox, Schiff, & Najdowski 2010).

Having recognized the importance of parental involvement, we should stress that the available empirical studies have mainly observed and measured the effectiveness of ABA-based interventions, in which the role of the caregiver was given little to no attention. Taking this into account, other studies, not focused on eating disorders, have analysed the effectiveness of an intervention in which parents were actively involved. An example of this is the study by Puliafico, Comer, and Albano (2013), who described an intervention aimed at reducing anxiety in two phases: in the first phase, the therapist trained the parents in using reinforcing behaviours which differed from their typical approach; in the second phase, the therapist worked with the child and the parents during the moment when approaching the anxiogenic stimulus (the CALM programme; Coaching Approach Behaviour and Leading by Modelling; 2013).

A form of intervention is starting to take shape in which cognitive/behavioural elements and parental involvement assume a central role, together with the possibility of conducting empirical studies to test its effectiveness in cases of eating disorders in developing individuals. Notably, and of relevance to the persistence of the beneficial effects of treatment, many scientific reports have emphasized how child representations tied to food rejection or aversion have rarely been considered, compared to the greater attention reserved to behavioural and cognitive techniques of desensitization and reinforcement. In an article published in the *Infant Mental Health Journal* (2007), Solter writes: "Treatment modalities for traumatic stress disorder that rely on exposure to traumatic themes through symbolic representations (such as language, images, or symbolic play) are therefore inappropriate for infants under 12 months of age" (p. 79).

Therefore, we need to consider how different techniques could integrate elements coming from different theories and how, according to age at onset and treatment, they could take into consideration the elaboration of the child's representational world, i.e., of the child's internal world.

Along with recent scientific evidence of infants' memory and cognition, attachment theory helps us understand some of the reasons behind behavioural approaches and their limited effectiveness. It also informs us about possible therapeutic alternatives that include working on the children's subjective experience and not just their objective one. In 1988, Winnicott wrote: "It is not possible to take for granted that the infant's psyche will form satisfactorily in partnership with the soma [...], psychosomatic life is an achievement" (p. 12).

Behavioural treatments focus on the exterior aspects of behaviour, bypassing the meaning that eating and the specific behaviour have for an individual as indicators of an intra-psychic conflict that is reflected on the food and that can have serious repercussions on emotional functioning and increase the risk of future relapse. Attachment theory, in fact, offers a framework to think about feeding interactions and dyadic relationships, conceptualizing the relationship children have with food and their relationship with the environment/world.

Eating involves the negotiation of the link between "inside and outside" and the importance of evaluating and facing relational issues (such as for example, the attachment types present in diagnostic subtypes of eating disorders) is often recognized as central to the possibility of changing dysfunctional eating patterns (Benoit et al. 2000; Chatoor 2009; Daws 1997; de Campora et al., 2019; Emanuel 2010).

The evaluation – which will be discussed in depth later – must in fact take into account the maternal emotional availability, the child's comfort/reassurance seeking behaviours, and the mother's responsiveness. What is "served", for example, with maternal milk becomes part of the inner world of the children, characterizing their behaviour towards food: anxiety, depression, frustration, as well as the mother's accuracy in the perception of eating behaviours, of the child's physical and emotional development, of the child's intentionality, and the negotiation of important issues such as dependence and autonomy. When new food is introduced from the outside (for example, when solids are introduced for the first time), potentially representing both a positive novelty and a source of fear, children need a secure base, an external source capable of regulating their state – regardless of whether that is doubt or open distress – in order to be able to resume exploration, and strengthen the transition to new eating patterns.

Considering attachment theory, certain guiding principles should be kept in mind and integrated into the treatment: many recommendations are already present in literature, even though they have not been explicitly articulated, discussed, and proposed inside a comprehensive and attachment-informed theoretical model. Any kind of problem in the dyadic relationship between mother and child that concerns the feeling of safety and/or the autonomy of the child, as well as the experiences of infant attachment organized in the adolescent mind, must be confronted in a systematic way, recognizing and working on these relational elements, on the child's mental organization in relation to the hunger and satiety stimuli, and, ultimately, on the child's regulatory abilities.

2. Mindful Emotion Regulation – Approach (MER-A): reading model and intervention on the ED in children and adolescents

The mindfulness-based approach is increasingly used in the treatment of a wide variety of pathologies (Allen, Chambers, & Knight 2006; Baer 2003). Mindfulness-based interventions are based on the ability to focus on the present moment, adopting a non-judgemental attitude. In fact, the ability to observe one's own thoughts, emotions, and physical sensations without evaluating their importance and truthfulness, and without trying to modify or avoid them, allows subjects to increase their awareness and, consequently, to opt for adaptive choices (Baer 2003; Kabat-Zinn 1990).

This approach has been used successfully in the treatment of eating disorders. For example, a recent version (Telch, Agras, & Linehan 2000) of Dialectical Behaviour Therapy (DBT; Linehan 1993) included the learning of mindfulness skills as a therapeutic target. More specifically, the main idea was that the ability to reflect in a non-judgemental way upon one's own actions would lead to a reduction or a cessation of those dysfunctional eating behaviours that prevailed because of negative emotional states. Many studies have recognized that difficulties in regulating emotions can cause and contribute to the persistence of eating disorders. One example of this is given by looking at binge eating behaviours as attempts to escape from emotional states that are too intense, or as unadaptive strategies aimed at reducing the impact of conditions that impose too much emotional pressure. These two theories are backed up by a large amount of empirical and clinical literature and are increasingly attracting interest. They have greatly contributed to the understanding of the mechanisms that govern our mental functions and to the study of different treatment trajectories. Even though mindfulness and emotional regulation are partly overlapping (Chambers, Gullone, & Allen 2009) – in fact one of the objectives of mindfulness-based protocols is the improvement of adaptive regulatory abilities – not enough attention has been given to the conceptualization of an integrated theoretical model with practical implications for a variety of treatment possibilities and that we could call the "Mindful Emotion Regulation – Approach".

This model is based on the need to include the different elements that comprise the clinical picture of the "here and now" of the disorder manifestation, which is extremely important in dealing with developing individuals. In this population, it is fundamental to observe different but coexisting aspects of eating, that is, to evaluate individual competencies and relational contexts that are very different and difficult to generalize about. One clear example is food rejection and its affective/relational meaning, as well as its cognitive effects on preschool children and their families, compared to the meaning of the same behaviour when seen in adolescence. The possibility of proposing an integrated model that is based both on mindfulness and on regulatory competencies requires, first of all, the recognition of the affective and cognitive components that eating is affected by.

In fact, in the presence of an eating disorder, we can observe both the adoption of an unadaptive behavioural sequence toward food (more or less rigid, depending on the age of the subject), and the presence of an emotional nucleus that often represents the original cause of the symptom. These perspectives have a strong impact on the techniques and on the interventions that can be adopted to deal with food disorders, as well as on their objectives. For example, therapies based on cognitivist theory aim at modifying the content of the events both cognitively and emotionally. This method is antecedent-focused, and therefore seeks to modify the unadaptive behavioural sequence from its outset. Other approaches, instead more based on mindfulness, seek to modify the *relationship* with those same events, by promoting a response-focused strategy, aimed at stimulating new ways of relating to potentially stressful situations and events.

The different phases of development, from birth to adolescence, paint a picture of each historical moment in the family's life, in which food represents the chosen means of communication. The clinician must therefore pay special attention, considering the many components at play, in order to promote, in the family, an accepting and non-judgemental attitude, capable of adequately controlling those emotions that emerge and accompany the manifestation of the symptom.

3. Conclusions

Interventions centred on mindfulness and focused on emotional regulation processes are increasingly being applied to a greater number of issues and disorders. Because of this, the development of a construct which includes both of these components would seem to be of great importance in order to tailor the design of the treatment according to the age of the subjects and their phase of development. The proposal of a Mindful Emotion Regulation – Approach represents an attempt to enable individuals to remain "present" throughout the meal, recognizing their changing emotional states and gaining the ability to regulate them. Thus, the individual can transition from an immediate reaction caused by particularly activating stimuli, to the ability to focus on the "here and now", even before concentrating on the content of the moment itself or of the task being performed.

This treatment methodology represents the common theme of all the interventions presented in the following chapters. Even though different disorders and developmental phases are treated with different clinical approaches, they all converge towards a conscious focus on recognizing emotions, with the shared objective of creating a mindful context around eating experiences.

Highlights

- Because of the multiplicity of factors involved in the etiopathogenesis of eating disorders, *a biopsychosocial approach* should be considered. The problems surrounding this type of approach *are related to the age when the symptoms appear.*

- Attachment theory helps us understand some of the reasons behind behavioural approaches and it also informs us about possible therapeutic alternatives that include working on the children's subjective experience. Attachment theory, in fact, offers a framework to think about feeding interactions and dyadic relationships, conceptualizing the relationship children have with food and their relationship with the environment/ world.
- Mindfulness-based interventions are based on the ability to focus on the present moment, adopting a non-judgemental attitude. In fact, the ability to observe one's own thoughts, emotions, and physical sensations without evaluating their importance and truthfulness, and without trying to modify or avoid them, allows subjects to increase their awareness and, consequently, to opt for adaptive choices.
- Many studies have recognized that difficulties in regulating emotions can cause and contribute to the persistence of eating disorders. One example of this is given by looking at binge eating behaviours as attempts to escape from emotional states that are too intense, or as unadaptive strategies aimed at reducing the impact of conditions that impose too much emotional pressure.
- Even though mindfulness and emotional regulation are partly overlapping, not enough attention has been given to the conceptualization of an integrated theoretical model with practical implications for a variety of treatment possibilities and that we could call "Mindful Emotion Regulation – Approach".
- Mindful Emotion Regulation – Approach is an integrated model that is based both on mindfulness and on regulatory competencies and requires, first of all, the recognition of the affective and cognitive components that eating is affected by.

Part II

Assessment and treatment across the life course

Overweight and obesity risk in the first three years of life

Gaia de Campora and Giulio Cesare Zavattini

1. Overweight – from the perinatal phase to the first three years of life: state of the art, research prospects, and prevention

Childhood obesity has become an epidemic in most Western Countries. Many studies have tried to investigate the risk factors for the development of excess weight and obesity and, from the available literature, it is possible to trace several factors in the aetiology of this disorder.

As suggested in some of these studies, early exposure to overfeeding or underfeeding, the quality of pre- and perinatal eating practices, and child development in general, play a fundamental role in the onset of obesity and in the development of disorders associated with it (i.e., diabetes and cardio-respiratory issues). Despite many studies having focused on the early risk factors for child obesity, the pathogenic mechanism is not yet clear. The available data point to the importance of understanding the underlying factors that lead to this condition, to track down the different pathways for the onset and progression of excess weight.

The general estimate is that in Europe 135 million citizens are overweight and/or obese. Among children and adolescents, there is an exponential growth in the overweight population, with one out of four children considered obese. The evaluation of excess weight during development has been the object of considerable debate in the attempt to adopt flexible measures that are appropriate for the specific population and transversal in relation to international studies.

During childhood and adolescence, the Body Mass Index (BMI) changes according to age and gender and in relation to these, specific cut-offs have been established to define overweight and obesity. BMI percentiles for example have been defined and used, based on international standards, especially those of the International Obesity Task Force (IOTF; Cole, Bellizzi, Flegel, & Dietz 2000), the World Health Organization (WHO 2006) and Must, Dallal and Dietz (MDD; 1991).[1] When percentiles were calculated using the IOTF methodology, the prevalence of excess weight was lower than what emerged using the other systems, with the IOTF method also showing a clear difference between childhood and adolescence (Wang 2004). Al-Sendi, Shetty and Musaiger (2003) completed a systematic comparison of the above-mentioned reference standards using 546 subjects between 12 and 17 years of age. The results showed that there was no considerable difference between IOTF and MDD, while there was a significant difference when utilizing the WHO system. Today, it is fairly common to speak in terms of BMI (the relationship between weight in kilos and height squared) even in instances of excess weight during development. There are three approaches for the categorization of BMI: (1) the more traditional one defines risk as being two standard deviations above average, (2) the new IOTF proposal which utilizes the BMI classifications normally used for adults, and (3) the standard set proposed by the Centers for Disease Control and Prevention (CDC; Kucmarski et al. 2000), which specifies obesity as being at or above the 95th percentile for BMI (Ogden, Carroll, & Flegal 2003). With reference to the CDC system, some studies have demonstrated that the same percentile attributed to children of different heights but of the same age represented clearly uneven weights. This observation would entail the need for a stratification of values based on height. Instead of proposing such a measurement, we evaluated the BMI – as is done with adults – running comparisons according to the different populations and applying these calculations to children between 5 and 18 years of age. Criteria have in fact been established to enable the alignment of the BMI of children with that of adults (Reilly 2002). This choice was made because of the ease in data measurement, because of the weak association with height, and because of the good precision with which it identifies the presence of body fat (Krebs et al. 2007). In this case, the percentile is associated with the child's gender and age, but not with the child's state of health. Therefore, children are considered "obese" when their BMI is higher than 30 or higher than the 95th percentile, depending on gender and age; while they are considered "overweight" when between the 85th and 95th percentile and between 25 and 30 BMI. On the other hand, for children under two years of age, it is usual to avoid descriptions of obesity or overweight, even though the supine body weight can be calculated according to the growth curve and can be predictive of obesity risk when it increases rapidly.

The most recent studies have, however, tried to add an interdisciplinary perspective to these biological perspectives, taking into account the reciprocal influences of the different factors. In fact, excess weight and obesity can be explained only partially by genetic factors, as shown by studies conducted on identical twins, which showed that genes only explained a small part of the variance of this phenomenon. Various authors (Agras & Mascola 2005; Whitaker 2011) have in fact stressed the importance of the intrauterine and perinatal phases of life as times when one can track dysfunctional eating patterns.[2] In this regard, pregnancy would seem to represent an ideal time to initiate an investigation on early risk factors. Women's weight before and during pregnancy has a strong influence on the child's health at birth. In particular, the BMI range seen in women during pregnancy indicates different risk trajectories for the infant. Specifically, a BMI below the norm contributes to a delay in foetal development and increases the likelihood of preterm delivery and of developing anaemia because of iron deficiency. On the other hand, a BMI above the norm (>25) is associated with different complications before and after delivery, including the development of gestational diabetes, preeclampsia, infertility, pregnancy-induced hypertension, foetal macrosomia (>4500 g), a substantial risk of caesarean delivery, and postpartum anaemia.

The above-mentioned risks are mainly tied to bio-medical consequences of being overweight during pregnancy. There are, however, risk factors associated with prenatal eating habits and with being overweight during pregnancy that appear to contribute to explaining the development of excess weight in the infant. For example, many studies have established an association between smoking during pregnancy and later obesity. The studies report that cigarette smoke is initially related to low birthweight, followed by a gradual increase in BMI (von Kries, Toschke, Koletzko, & Slikker 2002). Maternal smoking during pregnancy seems to affect the development of the infant's cerebral pathways connected to learning and to reward behaviours. The alteration of these functions would lead to poor impulse control, including overeating.

Shank et al. (2015) report how a tendency to lose control in front of food is noticeable from childhood, and leads to uninhibited and compulsive eating behaviours, that are the basis of overweight and obesity. In line with these studies, Tanofsky-Kraff, Marcus, Yanovski, and Yanovski (2008; Tanofsky-Kraff et al. 2014) have proposed a diagnostic classification – *Loss of Control – Eating Disorder* (LOC-ED) – applicable to children between 6 and 12 years of age. This classification includes impulsivity, resorting to food in the absence of hunger, and a psychological state of haziness, states that can be related to Binge Eating Disorder (BED), which can be diagnosed in adolescence, thus representing the psychopathological continuation of a condition that started earlier in life.

Numerous studies have pointed out the important role of breastfeeding in preventing childhood obesity. Both the lack of, or a shortened duration of breastfeeding appears to be frequently associated with childhood overweight/obesity. According to a retrospective and intergenerational perspective, this is evidenced by the fact overweight mothers themselves resort to breastfeeding less frequently and for a shorter time than average (< six months). The reasons leading to a decrease in breastfeeding in overweight and obese women are not yet clear (Baker, Michaelsen, Rasmussen, & Sørensen 2004; Baker, Michaelsen, Sørensen, & Rasmussen 2007; Li, Jewell, & Grummer-Strawn 2003; Mehta, Siega-Riz, Herring, Adair, & Bentley 2011; Oddy et al. 2006). On the other hand, it is very clear that there is a protective effect of breastfeeding against the risk of developing obesity and excess weight (Arenz, Rückerl, Koletzko, & von Kries 2004; Harder, Bergmann, Kallischnigg, & Plagemann 2005; Owen, Martin, Whincup, Smith, & Cook 2005; Weden, Brownell, & Rendall 2012). The empirical evidence seems to point to protective mechanisms in breastfeeding, although the available studies are not in complete agreement on this. Among the explanations with more support, there is the different caloric content between formula and breast milk. Other studies have stressed the behavioural aspect of breastfeeding, which acts as a "hunger regulator". The process occurring inside the mother–child dyad during breastfeeding revolves around the behaviour of the infants and their satiety signal. The mother is not able to determine the quantity of milk offered by her breasts, therefore her attention will be focused on the child's request and interest in the food or on the child's satiety signal (DiSantis, Hodges, Johnson, & Fisher 2011; Farrow & Blissett 2006; Taveras, Rifas-Shiman, Scanlon, Grummer-Strawn, Sherry, & Gillman 2006; Wright, Fawcett, & Crow 1980). On the other hand, the quantity of formula that is offered depends completely on the mother's cognition and choices. In this way, children are given a more passive receptive role which could potentially stimulate them less in recognizing their own internal signals.

The literature presented here not only underlines the tendency toward an intergenerational transmission of overweight/obesity, but also points out the importance of the regulatory processes that are established in the feeding interactions and inside the dyadic relationship between mother and child (de Campora & Meldolesi, 2014).

2. Prevention starts with the relationship: the use of video feedback at home

Preventative strategies aimed at avoiding child overweight and obesity clearly represent the ideal one should strive towards. As of today, there are no standardized guidelines that help us in this, but there are numerous recommendations that encourage good daily practices which improve the child's health following birth. In cases where the adoption of these best practices proves challenging, the key question to ask is "how can we promote health to prevent child overweight from the perinatal stage?" As examples, we will describe several strategies that can be easily adopted by practitioners who deal with prenatal and perinatal care, and then we will describe our approach.

Barnett (1995) lists five possible strategies to prevent the occurrence of disorders during the perinatal phase: (1) discuss with future parents their feelings of adequacy vs. inadequacy in their role as parents; (2) facilitate as much as possible the transition to parenthood, promoting self-reliance and keeping stress, anxiety, and symptoms of depression within a reasonable range; (3) recognize those who are at risk of mood disorders or other pathologies; (4) actively intervene with those who display a clear clinical condition; (5) recognize and support those who are at risk of becoming *fragile* parents, because of their own vulnerability or because of temperamental and/or individual aspects of the child. The first approach to consider is therefore definitely informational. Information acts as prevention in and of itself, and in order to play this role, it needs to reach those requiring intervention. This aspect must be enriched and integrated with the possibility of providing a support network around the mother–child dyad, activating modalities of communication that reinforce competencies and aimed at problem-solving, supporting, at the same time, the exploration of the parental experience.

Along these prevention pathways, a series of possible early interventions could be added for families that show an above-average risk of developing perinatal disorders and/or psychopathological conditions. Early interventions include home visiting (Olds & Kitzman 1990; Olds et al. 1997), supporting pre-term babies, and psychotherapy for women with high levels of anxiety and post-partum depressive/psychotic disorders. The summary table showed below reports the synthesis of the empirical studies that dealt with interventions in the perinatal period.

In addition, more recent literature documents the use of Video-feedback Intervention to Promote Positive Parenting (VIPP), which is a useful tool to offer early support and to actively help the dyads at risk. The value of using VIPP is the possibility for direct access to the mother–child interaction, without having to rely on the parents' reports. The specific objective of VIPP is to increase the mother's responsiveness and to help create a safe context for the attachment bond (Bakermans-Kranenburg, van Ijzendoorn, & Juffer 2003). This type of intervention is most effective if it is introduced in the first year of life. During this developmental phase, particularly in the case of first-time mothers, caregivers are more likely to accept advice and suggestions for issues they are facing for the first time. In these situations, the family routine has not yet been established and the problems are still new and transient.

VIPP, as created by Juffer, Bakermans-Kranenburg, and Van IJzendoorn (2008), has these essential objectives: (1) to promote the parents' ability to pay attention to the signals and needs expressed by the child; (2) to help the parents develop observation and empathy; (3) to reinforce the positive behaviours adopted by the parents, especially those that evidence sensitivity towards the child; and (4) to engage the parents in a dialogue about their past attachment experiences and about the possible influence these might be having on their relationship with their child. VIPP was in fact created to help struggling parents take a step back with respect to the emotional spiral in which they and the child find themselves, examining what emerges and observing the interactions from a different point of view. The procedure can vary in its application, but fundamentally uses two main approaches (Bakermans-Kranenburg, van Ijzendoorn, & Juffer 2003; Fukkink 2008; Juffer & Steele 2014). In the first approach, the use of video feedback focuses on (1) behaviour and the gateway into the relationship is based on the interactions and behaviours observed within the dyad (Stern, 1985, 2004). In this case, the use of video recording helps maintain the focus on the here and now (e.g., McDonough 2005). In the second approach, the focus is on (2) the mother's mental representations of herself, of the child, and of their relationship, as gateway for intervention. In this case, video recording is used to gain quicker access into the mother's early experiences (Lieberman 2004). The distinction between these two approaches is not always clear and, in some cases, a combined approach is used (Beebe 2003; Cramer 1998; Egeland, Weinfeld, Bosquet, & Cheng 2000).

In summary, within VIPP the focus remains on the meaningful and real events occurring in the dyadic relationship, avoiding the use of judgements, even if positive, and avoiding direct attempts aimed at changing behaviours. The result of this type of approach leads to an awareness of the dynamics of the relationship and to a maturational process of thought, that we could call "mindful".

In our clinical practice, as will later be shown with a clinical example, we adopt a VIPP procedure that has been adapted to the context of perinatal eating disorders and, more specifically, to the risk of intergenerational transmission of overweight. The research of Stein et al. (2006) is the only study we know of that used this approach in a systematic way, adapting it to the perinatal diet. From this starting point, we concentrated on the need to prevent the conflict that characterizes meals, focusing our observations on the emotional exchange between mother and child, as a means to producing new knowledge on the relational context. Our protocol includes 12 meetings: six of these are dedicated to video-recording meals at home, and in the remining six, using footage from the previous recordings, the mother's behaviours and those of her child are observed and reflected upon, together with the mother. The video recording takes place every other meeting, while during the observation/dialogue meeting, the focus is gradually shifted towards certain fundamental relational behaviours. Specifically, there are three central steps: (1) keeping the children's perspective in mind, focusing on the signals they give; (2) confronting the parents' perspective, emphasizing the moments of mutual exchange, sharing, and emotional tuning within the dyad; (3) promoting in the mother the exploration of those behaviours that, according to her, represent "signals of conflict in relation to food".

The case of Sara and Matteo will now be described, keeping in mind the characteristics of video-feedback interventions in the perinatal period.

3. Sara and Matteo: a story of "power"

The first time we met Sara and Giacomo, they were pregnant with Matteo, their second born. It was during the third trimester in the pregnancy. In collaboration with the Department of Obstetrics and Gynaecology of a hospital in Rome, we provide a comprehensive evaluation of the mother's psychological and emotional status, and we offer the possibility of support to all women who face a high-risk pregnancy. We also offer post-partum support and assistance in those cases that we believe show the possibility of perinatal risk. In these cases, our support can last up to one year and is conducted at the family's home.

Sara had a relatively peaceful pregnancy, with the only risk being possibly developing gestational diabetes, which actually did not happen. Sara had in fact a long history of being overweight, even before pregnancy, which had become worse over time. During her gynaecological visits, she was told to follow a healthy diet, because her condition could have led to a series of complications and negative outcomes both for her and for Matteo, including early delivery, caesarean section, pre-eclampsia, and foetal macrosomia. In spite of the attentive care of the medical staff and in spite of our attempts to make her explore the causes of this behaviour and its possible consequences, Sara almost completely ignored the indications she had received, gaining weight, and exceeding the prescribed ranges during each trimester.[3] As a consequence, Sara's blood pressure greatly increased, and she delivered Matteo by C-section. Matteo was born a healthy baby but very close to being diagnosed with macrosomia, with a birthweight of 9.2 pounds (4.2 kilos).

With this in mind, we offered Sara and Giacomo post-partum support.[4] Sara's behaviour, of which eating represented a single element, seemed to be characterized by difficulties in impulse control and poor sensibility in taking care of Matteo, since before his birth.

One month after they went home, we contacted Sara, who described a "wonderful baby, who sleeps, lets me sleep, and breastfeeds without any problems". She also told us that Giacomo would have to travel on business and would be gone for a few months. We therefore set up a meeting before Giacomo's departure, in order to inform both parents of the process we would follow. Sara, however, kept postponing the meeting until after the husband's departure, an event that appeared to trigger a depressive reaction in her. Then, she contacted us to agree on a date to meet, reporting somatic problems and an "insurmountable" tiredness.

We finally succeeded in meeting Sara and Matteo. We immediately noticed that the mother's mind was completely absorbed in her own physical and psychological ailments, appearing to almost "forget" about Matteo and Margherita (her first born). Matteo seemed to be facilitating his mother and her needs by being surprisingly calm even when awake and hungry. Six-year-old Margherita was showing a slight speech impairment, on the background of emerging depressive states.[5] We briefly presented our procedure, but we postponed the beginning of the home visits to the following week. Sara, however, contacted us, again cancelling the appointment. In the following four weeks, she periodically contacted us to postpone the meetings with different excuses, but still "compulsively" talking about herself. We then decided to keep the telephone contacts, trying to offer a space that could welcome her need to be listened to, but with precise time limits to it. Our impression was in fact that Sara had a strong need for closeness, but was also very scared by it, as partly seen in the somatic complaints[6] that followed her separation from her husband.

Six months later, it seemed Sara was ready to start the home visits and we met again. Matteo was eight months old and he was at the 85th percentile in the growth curve, an element of risk for developing overweight/obesity. During this meeting, Sara described a baby who "cries constantly for no reason", who "never behaves well", and who "fusses when I feed him". Sara was convinced that Matteo's main problem was his obstinate and irritable personality. This did not seem to cause eating problems, like rejection or selectivity of food, but it created a conflicting emotional environment, which was too difficult for Sara to manage on her own.

After this "new first meeting", Sara contacted us again, saying that "this commitment is too much" for her at that moment and that she felt "too tired to be able to go through with it". The prolonged absence of her husband during a trying time like the post-partum phase removed a fundamental source of support from her, increasing her sense of isolation and her depressive states. Unlike in the previous interruption, Sara was able to speak the truth about the reason she wanted to stop the meetings, leading us to believe that the relationship we had started was based on greater trust and on our flexibility in negotiating the right distances to keep.

For the next year and a half, Sara continued to contact us, without a specific schedule or routine, but keeping us always up to date about Matteo's growth, and describing him again as a "good well-behaved baby, who does not cause any problems".

In the meanwhile, Giacomo returned definitively home. Sara contacted us saying that she was ready to start the process with us, because Matteo had become "difficult" again. In light of our previous meetings and of the information we had gathered along the way, we proposed the video feedback intervention to Sara, hoping that this would give us a more immediate access to the conflict within the dyad, and would offer Sara a perspective through which to observe her relationship with her son.

Matteo, over two years of age, was showing the beginnings of overweight, which immediately reminded us of his relationship with Sara since pregnancy. We observed the feeding interactions, and the most striking element was the conflict between mother and child, which manifested itself in the form of protest. Matteo did not cry during these episodes, but he showed a strong opposition to the mother's presence. Sara tried her best to feed Matteo and to seem adequate in our presence, but her sense of frustration was evident, as was the fact that the exchange we were observing was not the escalation of a problem within the dyad, but the consolidation of an emotional pattern that was reflected in many areas, of which eating was only one.

During our next meeting, thanks to the father's assistance, we reserved a moment to watch with Sara an excerpt of the video recording. Right away, it was clear that the mother was struggling to understand the meaning of Matteo's protest, beyond its immediate manifestation. Sara's answers related to Matteo going *against* Sara, throwing almost vindictive tantrums. We found this explanation very interesting because it attributed a very subtle emotional process to Matteo, pointing us towards the hypothesis that Sara had been unknowingly treating Matteo, in the absence of his father, "like a little adult", capable of plotting against his mother. We thus decided to keep our focus on this aspect: *why was Matteo protesting?* We tried to use our next two meetings to explore this question, observing Sara feeding Matteo, how Matteo responded to this, and how Sara reacted to Matteo's behaviour. We tried to construct a logical chain of actions, in which we could see the connection between cause and effect, creating a space where Sara was free to take time and observe her son's emotional expressions and their meaning, claiming back that time she felt she could not enjoy any longer, because of the continuous escalation of anger. Gradually, this space enabled the mother to mainly gain the emotional predisposition to notice different aspects in Matteo's lunch experience. Tenderness, curiosity, distractions, and the relationship with his sister emerged. Sara started seeing Matteo as a child, making space for thoughts about his "needs", and her role as regulator of them.

When we realized that Sara had brought her relationship with Matteo as the central element of our process, we shifted the focus on the *meaning of their behaviours at that moment.* Our objective was in fact to promote, in the mind of the mother, a focus on the present moment that could then be transferred to all their future interactions, enabling her to observe and listen to what is *really* happening, without fear of mistakes[7] or of being judged by the presence of a "competent" female. At the end of our eighth meeting, Sara told us that she had noticed how Matteo assumed a specific posture right before she showed him the spoon and started feeding him. In fact, Matteo stiffened, clenched his fists, and when the spoon was in his mouth, he banged his hands on the table. Why? What did this sequence mean? In the following meetings, Sara reflected and shared her observations with us, gradually moving from the *here and now* to a dimension of temporal reconstruction, that could include all family members.

After this important passage, Sara began to be more empathetic towards Matteo's protests, loosening those behaviours that previously led her to hand-feed Matteo, instead granting him more freedom to touch, to play, and to try to eat on his own. As a result of this enhanced maternal availability and sensibility, Matteo started showing a wider range of emotions, more positive, which, even though still occurring in-between moments of irritability, were enough to reinforce Sara's growing desire to take care of her son. Meals began lasting longer, in order to allow Matteo to perform the routine with autonomy. This change also altered Matteo's regulatory abilities, and by the end of our meetings, he had started to interrupt the meal signalling his satiety.

4. Conclusions

The elements that characterize the risk for perinatal eating disorders can be divided into two categories: a familiar history of conflicted relationships with food, of an emotional/psychological nature, and/or problems tied to medical/

biological conditions that hinder the normal development of eating habits. In the first case, situations such as a history of maternal eating disorders, a poor or completely absent support network, or a particularly difficult or irritable infant temperament, can exponentially increase the possibility that meals become times of confrontation, rather than togetherness (de Campora et al., 2016).

The case that we presented shows a powerful combination of different elements. Sara had created the idea in her mind, since pregnancy, of a child who would not cause problems regardless of the situation. In fact, at the time Sara was facing two important separations, one from the husband and the other represented by Matteo's birth. In that moment, our presence represented the threat of another possible separation and presented the risk of appearing fragile or inadequate in front of strangers. Her husband's return home made her feel like she had found her place inside a family – she no longer was the only one doing all the work, but simply one of the parents. This change in the family organization was easily understandable for Sara, but Matteo needed a time and a place to metabolize the new situation. The food exchange between Matteo and his mother had thus become the battlefield for exercising the power that had been abruptly taken away from him. Because of the difficulties showed by Matteo, Sara tried to feed him, limiting his fussing as much as possible. But this only exacerbated the conflict, because it was pushing Matteo (almost three years old, at the time) towards a dependent relationship with his mother. Conflict therefore seemed to be the only instrument Matteo had to communicate the paradoxical phase he was living: he was big enough to share "his spaces" with a stranger (the father), but at the same time he was to be so little as to need spoon-feeding, instead of experimenting with what he could and wanted to do. This dichotomy Matteo was living through seemed to correspond exactly to Sara's descriptions during our phone conversations: a child who was alternatively described as good or bad, easy or difficult, devoid of any nuances and without any possibility of being present in the mother's mind as a combination of these qualities.

Certainly, Matteo's excess weight represented the result of an environment *in utero* that was predisposed to this condition, but it also reflected the mother/son relationship from the beginning. In this relationship, Matteo was not seen as a child expressing needs, therefore he adjusted along the lines of the paradoxical messages he was receiving: I rebel, but I keep eating.

The reiteration of similar situations leads the child to a sense of confusion – included among the diagnostic criteria of LOC-ED – in which emotions prevail and the food is assimilated in a way that is not connected with actual hunger. In these cases, eating is not the answer to a nutritional need, but the means or the context in which to communicate distress within a relationship.

The procedure we briefly described here seems appropriate because it prioritizes a focus on the present moment. This not only promotes an active involvement on the part of the caregiver, but it also shows that the relationship between mother and child is a process in continuous evolution. If one of the two changes, the other changes as well, establishing a rhythm based on reciprocal exchanges and on the effects that each partner has on the other, in an attempt to regulate the emotional exchange, in addition to the food exchange.

Highlights

- Early exposure to overfeeding or underfeeding, the quality of pre- and perinatal eating practices, and child development in general, play a fundamental role in the onset of obesity and in the development of disorders associated with it.
- Excess weight and obesity can be explained only partially by genetic factors, as shown by studies conducted on identical twins. Various authors have in fact stressed the importance of the intrauterine and perinatal phases of life as times when one can track dysfunctional eating patterns.
- The literature presented not only underlines the tendency toward an intergenerational transmission of overweight/obesity, but also points out the importance of the regulatory processes that are established in the feeding interactions and inside the dyadic relationship between mother and child.
- Preventative strategies aimed at avoiding child overweight and obesity clearly represent the ideal one should strive towards. Along these prevention pathways, a series of possible early interventions could be added for families that show an above-average risk, and including home visiting, supporting pre-term babies, and psychotherapy for women with high levels of anxiety and post-partum depressive/psychotic disorders.
- Recent literature documents the use of Video-feedback Intervention to Promote Positive Parenting (VIPP), which is a useful tool to offer early support and to actively help the dyads at risk, increasing the mother's responsiveness and helping to create a safe context for the attachment bond. The result of this type of approach leads to an awareness of the dynamics of the relationship and to a maturational process of thought, that we could call *mindful*.
- We adapt the VIPP procedure to the context of perinatal eating disorders and, more specifically, to the risk of intergenerational transmission of overweight.

Notes

1 The IOTF parameters provide an age and gender adjustment based on the average values obtained from different populations. From these values cut-off points were established in order to determine which subjects were overweight or obese before 18 years of age. On the other hand, the WHO established the 85th percentile as the international norm for identifying subjects "at risk" of overweight between 10 and 19 years of age. In subjects under 10, the use of Z scores was recommended,

adjusted for weight and height. The MDD system relies instead on an ample collection of cases gathered by the US National Center for Health Statistics between 1971 and 1974, which records a range comprised between the 85th and the 95th percentile for children and teenagers at risk of being overweight.

2 The journal *Obesity: A Research Journal*, leader in the research on the causes of obesity, recently dedicated an entire issue (*It all starts in the womb*) to the subject of the influence of prenatal life on individuals' future weight.

3 In this regard, the Institute of Medicine (IOM 2009), in the face of a clear necessity, revised the criteria that had previously been published in 1999, on the basis of the BMI categories proposed by WHO, defining weight standards during gestation. In general, IOM recommends not to gain more than 1 or 2 kilos in the first trimester. For the following two trimesters, the recommendations vary according to pre-pregnancy BMI and they are the same as those adopted in Italy.

4 In this initial phase, we are referring to a home-based form of psychological support, as previously described, and not to a VIPP intervention yet.

5 We will not describe Margherita's issues and her relationship with her parents here, due to space constraints.

6 These in fact seemed to be a way of activating caregiving behaviours in others, without the need of explicitly asking for affection.

7 This is the central moment of the process and also the moment in which Sara was finding a balance between the idea of being a "victim" of the son and the risk of considering herself a bad mother (as an outcome of elaboration).

Chapter 4

Infantile anorexia and Post-Traumatic Feeding Disorder in early infancy

Loredana Lucarelli

I. Introduction

In the last few decades, developmental psychopathology has focused on a comprehensive study of the complex interactions between the biological, psychological and environmental process that may influence the differences among individuals, the developmental pathways (Sroufe 1990) and the possible normal or pathological outcomes (Cicchetti & Cohen 2006; Sameroff 2010).

The theoretical and research backgrounds of this scientific discipline are based on the developments of the theories of attachment and of inter-subjectivity and on Infant Research, which contributed to significantly altering our understanding of the developmental processes through which infants develop stable patterns of experimentation and adjustment to the environment, organizing and consolidating the attachment bonds with their caregivers.

A fundamental innovation was represented by the hypothesis of an early structuring of the psychic world, of the possibility of tracing in new-borns, from the first weeks of life, an innate social intelligence that makes them ready to interact with their partners (*proto-conversational readiness*, Trevarthen & Aitken 2001), the minds of new-borns, that is, already being organized in a dialogic way from birth.

This predisposition is, however, not supposed to be enough to guarantee the development of the infant's abilities, without the support of early interactions with caregivers (Papoušek 2007; Stern 1995). The innate motivation (*primary activity* (Sander 2007)) towards seeking relationships and towards reaching a relational reciprocity would therefore constitute a necessary, but insufficient, condition for the development and integration of communicative abilities. The initiatives and reactions of the caregivers, experimented during communicative exchanges, become a constant in the interactive environment for the new-born, distinctive elements of the processes of micro-regulation activated to adjust reciprocal interactions; the coherence and predictability of affects and of the infant's socio-communicative repertoire develop through these processes of micro-regulation in primary care (Stern 2010).

The system of affective communication between caregiver and infant has been defined as an intersubjective matrix (Stern 2004) and a self-regulation system (Sander 2007), that is a fundamental context of development in which the individual can express personal motivations co-constructing relational models that contribute to self-definition. The ability to take into consideration one's own mental states and those of others emerges from the early inter-subjective experiences between caregivers and infants, particularly from the predictable experience of being recognized and understood in one's own mental and intentional states.

The developmental acquisition of this intrapsychic and interpersonal ability is fundamental in influencing the modulation and the regulation of affective and mental states: the experiences that are recognized and understood can in fact be integrated, contained and safeguarded in the mind without the defensive distortion of experience and of the affects connected to it (Fonagy, Gergely, Jurist, & Target 2002; Slade, 2010). In this regard, research and clinical work on mind-mindedness (Meins et al. 2002) – that is the recognition by parents of the intentional and mental states of their own infant – and on the reflective function of parents – that is their ability to reflect on their own internal mental experience and that of their own infant, in terms of intentions, motivations and feelings of the other (Slade 2010), and the connected experiences of empathic attunement (Stern, 1995) – have explored the influence on the development of infant mentalization of this scaffolding context,[1] with which infants start to give meaning to their own behaviour, in terms of the underlying mental states. In relation to this, it has been shown that "non-reflective parents" tend to deny the existence of mental and affective states in themselves and in their children, focusing their attention instead on behaviour and behavioural problems, with no apparent interest in what the infant thinks or feels, overlooking the mental states and the affects that could be maintaining or eliciting the behaviour. In this condition, cycles of "non-mentalizing interactions" are soon established between caregiver and infant, tending towards repetition and reinforcement (Slade 2010).

Conversely, a healthy development of the attachment relationship is favoured by the presence of mental representations that can develop characteristics of flexibility, fluidity and coherence, which allow the parent to experience the full range of possible emotions and affects in the encounter with the infant, without the need to produce defensive mechanisms that distort affects and emotions (Rosenblum, Dayton, & McDonough 2006). In this way, parents will be able to effectively regulate their infant's affective experience, helping them give meaning to it, recognizing it as their own and sharing it with their interaction partners. At the same time, the parents will be able to sync with the peculiar and exclusive characteristics of their own infant, encouraging self-regulatory and assertive initiatives and supporting the unravelling of the "developmental paradox", which includes the two co-evolving poles of "being together with" and "being distinct from", that is, inter-subjectivity and disengagement from the other (Sander 1991, pp. 153–160; Winnicott 1965).

In the first months of the infant's life, a fundamental development task therefore consists precisely in the regulation of behaviours related to physiological homeostasis, that is the effectiveness of the caregiver and the child in establishing a dyadic regulation model that promotes nutrition, sleep and physical well-being, so that basic biological rhythms can become organized and stabilized. In particular, in order for adequate feeding to be achieved in relation to nutritional homeostasis (Chatoor 1996), the new-born must be able to reach a state of vigilance and calmness that might, instead, be particularly compromised by states of strong excitability, or excessive irritability, or of persistent sleepiness during early feeding, in which case feeding difficulties might begin in the neonatal period. A depressed or anxious mother may find it difficult to compensate for these dysfunctional characteristics of her child and to adapt her behaviour by trying to modulate the characteristics of the holding environment for her child; these mothers might instead react to the low responsiveness of their new-born by dysfunctionally increasing or reducing the stimulation necessary to improve the state of regulation during early feeding. Infants with an immature nervous system (babies who were immature or premature at birth), or with medical problems, such as early colic, or gastro-oesophageal reflux may be at risk for this disorder. The mother and the new-born show difficulties developing a relational reciprocity, and there is a risk of the clinical condition becoming persistent, with the possibility that a feeding disorder of reciprocity is established in the infant–caregiver relationship. Indeed, dyadic reciprocity normally begins to manifest itself between 2 and 4 months of the new-born's life, when the neonatal endogenous rhythms diminish in favour of an organization predominantly regulated by the affective and social interaction between mother and child. The time spent sleeping by the infant decreases, the waking time increases and the infant responds more readily to social stimuli, as highlighted by changes in the interactions, now characterized by reciprocated gaze, vocalizations and physical closeness, which are more and more mutually regulated. The reflexive cry of hunger is replaced by an intentional crying and by demand vocalizations and the infant communicates his state of satiety more clearly.

Subsequently, the developmental phase of "transition to autonomous nutrition" is a developmental task of the child and of the mother–child dyad, which typically starts after 6–9 months of life. In the gradual transition from weaning to being able to eat independently, these represent, in fact, turning points (Brazelton & Greenspan 2000) identified as critical periods of child development, during which almost all aspects of the relational functioning of children change, and their relationship with their parents must be reorganized in terms of the children's newly acquired emotional, cognitive and motor abilities. The parents' sensitive recognition of these patterns of exploration and experimentation supports the development of eating skills, of the internal regulation of hunger/satiety signals and of the affective process of separation-autonomy.

2. Relevant clinical aspects of the avoidant/restrictive food intake disorder: Infantile Anorexia and Post-Traumatic Feeding Disorder

Recently, in the latest edition of the Diagnostic and Statistical Manual of Mental Disorders (DSM-5; APA 2013), eating disorders are classified in a single section: "Feeding and Eating Disorders", in line with the recognition, in research and clinical work, of a psychopathological continuity of these disorders from infancy, to adolescence and adulthood, as evidenced by the DSM-5 Eating Disorders Work Group, which contributed to the writing of the DSM-5 (Bryant-Waugh, Markham, Kreipe, & Walsh 2010; Bryant-Waugh 2013). Specifically, however, in the "Feeding and Eating Disorders" section, the DSM-5 provides the diagnostic criteria for the "Avoidant/ Restrictive Food Intake Disorder" (ARFID) – which replaced the "Feeding and Eating Disorders of Infancy or Early Childhood" category, previously described in the DSM-IV.

In a recent editorial commenting on the potential of the DSM-5, James Leckman and Daniel Pine (2012) underlined that the nosological decision to remove the category of "Disorders Usually First Diagnosed in Infancy, Childhood or Adolescence" is generally considered a positive change, as is the detailed description of age-specific characteristics for each disorder, as it reflects the fact that "development" is now considered an essential dimension for most mental disorders, and its role is therefore included with greater prominence. Furthermore, Leckman and Pine underline how this change will pose a challenge to many clinicians who focus on the paediatric age, and how there will consequently be a need for specialized texts and a separate primary care classification system of development disorders, specifically built for clinicians working on the mental health of children and their families.

The ARFID category in the DSM-5 represents an important recognition of the empirical research and clinical work that has been carried out in recent decades in the field of childhood eating disorders. The ARFID category was in fact developed on the basis of the DC:0–3R (Zero-To-Three 2005) classification of childhood eating disorders.[2]

Specifically, Infantile Anorexia is the diagnostic subtype characterized by "apparent lack of interest in food or eating"; Sensory Food Aversions are the diagnostic subtype of avoidance based on the sensory characteristics of food; and the Feeding Disorder associated with a Gastrointestinal Tract Disorder, also called Post-Traumatic Feeding Disorder (PTFD) (Chatoor, Ganiban, Harrison, & Hirsch 2001), is the diagnostic subtype defined by fear and concerns about adverse oral and/or feeding experiences in the child's clinical history. Table 4.1 describes the DC:0–3R diagnostic criteria in relation to the relevant clinical conditions included in the DSM-5 ARFID category.

Table 4.1 Eating disorders between 0 and 3 years of age (Axis I: DC:0–3R, Zero To Three 2005, 2008)

Infantile Anorexia

1   Refuses to eat adequate amounts of food for at least 1 month.
2   The onset of the food refusal occurs before the third year of life.
3   Does not communicate hunger, lacks interest in food, but shows great interest toward either exploration or interaction with the caregiver, or both.
4   Shows significant growth deficiency.
5   The food refusal did not follow a traumatic event.
6   The food refusal is not due to an underlying medical illness.

Sensory Food Aversions

1   Consistently refuses to eat foods with specific tastes, textures and/or smells.
2   Onset of the food refusal occurs during the introduction of a new type of food (for example, may drink one type of milk but refuse another; may eat carrots but refuse green beans; may drink milk but refuse baby food).
3   Eats with no difficulty when offered preferred foods.
4   The food refusal may cause specific nutritional deficiencies or delays in oral motor development.

Feeding Disorder associated with a Gastrointestinal Tract Disorder

1   The food refusal follows a traumatic event or repeated traumatic insults to the oropharyngeal or gastrointestinal tract (for example, choking, severe vomiting, nasogastric or endotracheal intubation, aspirations) that trigger intense distress in the child.
2   Consistent refusal to eat, which may be manifested in one of the following ways:
    –   Refuses bottle but may accept feeding by spoon or hand
    –   Refuses solid foods but may accept the bottle
    –   Refuses all oral feedings
3   Reminders of the traumatic event(s) cause distress, as manifested in one or more of the following ways:
    –   May show anticipatory distress when positioned for feeding
    –   Shows intense resistance when approached with bottle or food
    –   Shows intense resistance to swallowing food that is placed in the mouth
4   The food refusal may represent an acute or chronic threat to the child's nutritional status.

A further innovation introduced by the ARFID category is the conceptualization of different diagnostic types of eating problems with both organic and non-organic components, the implementation of which proved challenging in research on the diagnosis and classification of childhood eating disorders (Bryant-Waugh & Piepenstock 2008). The clinical problem is relevant if one considers that childhood eating disorders are observed and evaluated in a wide variety of clinical contexts: general practitioners, gastroenterologists, language and motor therapists, child neuropsychiatrists, psychologists. A strict distinction between secondary eating disorders and those associated with medical problems, or functional deficiencies, or emotional and relational problems is often very difficult to make in clinical practice. Feeding problems in infancy can in fact present multiple components at their origin, or not infrequently feeding problems might persist in many children even when the organic cause has been addressed, as in Post-Traumatic Eating Disorders (PTED), highlighting the need for a multidisciplinary diagnostic and therapeutic approach (Bryant-Waugh, Markham, Kreipe, & Walsh 2010; Chatoor 2009).

In this chapter, the discussion will focus on two relevant clinical conditions, Infantile Anorexia and Post-Traumatic Eating Disorder.[3] In fact, while these conditions can be considered examples of different aetiologies at the origin of the developmental disorder, it will be shown how a common approach, useful in guiding clinical evaluation and treatment, addresses the quality of the emotional relationship with the caregivers.

The relevant clinical condition of Infantile Anorexia (see Table 4.1) (Chatoor 1996, 2009) is manifested through an intense and persistent refusal of food and a significant acute or chronic malnutrition of the child, which may have different levels of severity, often in relation to the nutritional developmental history of the child which, as previously discussed, may have been characterized by early relational mis-attunement between the caregiver and the child. Children with IA are described as very uninterested in food, almost always distracted by external stimuli and with a lack of appetite, which intensely worries parents, who feel powerless in facing the situation. Parents, especially mothers, emphasize the intense behavioural opposition of these children. The procedures these parents often put in place (distractions, games during meals, offers of different foods at different times outside of regular meal times, threats or coercions) do not have a significant effect on the amount of food ingested by the child, who progressively loses weight. The history of these children presents no oral and/or feeding traumatic experiences or medical conditions that may otherwise explain their disorder.

Infantile Anorexia (IA) represents the diagnostic subtype that has been most investigated by clinical research in recent years. The most explored variables are: the child's temperament and emotion regulation, mother–child interactions, and maternal psychopathology. Recent data also point towards taking into account the paternal parenting function and its influence on the clinical manifestation of IA and on the mother–child caregiving and co-parenting system (Atzaba-Poria et al. 2010; Lucarelli, Simonelli, & Ammaniti 2012).

Cross-sectional studies conducted on infants with IA, during the first two years of life, found temperament to be "difficult" compared to both *picky eaters* (infants who take food in a reduced manner, without reaching the level of severity of infants with IA), and control children with normal growth and regular feeding patterns (Ammaniti, Lucarelli, Cimino, D'Olimpio, & Chatoor 2010; Chatoor, Ganiban, Hirsh, Borman-Spurrell, & Mrazek 2000; Lucarelli,

Cimino, D'Olimpio, & Ammaniti 2013). According to these studies, the temperamental profile of children with IA presents difficulties in regulating and stabilizing basic biological rhythms (nutrition and sleep), higher levels of activity, negative social orientation and affectivity, and lower levels of positive affectivity. A study found a higher physiological level of arousal in a sample of infants with IA, during their second year of life, compared to a control group (Chatoor, Ganiban, Surles, & Doussard-Roosevelt 2004). Cross-sectional studies conducted with children aged 2–3 years, and longitudinal research conducted on children from infancy to school age, have further explored the emotional-behavioural functioning of children with clinical diagnosis of IA, highlighting both internalizing and externalizing problems in emotion regulation (Ammaniti, Lucarelli, Cimino, D'Olimpio, & Chatoor 2010, 2012; Lucarelli et al. 2013).

The difficult emotion regulation of these children shows continuity from infancy to school age, although the longitudinal study of children diagnosed with IA in the first three years of life, but with no significant clinical treatment, showed an improvement in malnutrition at the age of 5–7 in most children, with 10% of children still presenting a moderate degree of malnutrition in school age (Ammaniti et al. 2012). In this longitudinal study, however, an assessment of the quality of eating behaviour patterns in the children previously diagnosed with IA, and re-examined at school age, confirmed a continuity of significant behavioural difficulties related to nutrition. In particular, this research revealed a different developmental trajectory of eating patterns, compared to a control group paired by age and assessed longitudinally, showing that children, with a prior diagnosis of IA, had more dysfunctional scores in: *Satiety Responsiveness* (generally manifested through a limited food intake), *Lack of Enjoyment of Food* (lack of pleasure tied to eating and lack of interest in food), and *Food Fussiness* (idiosyncrasies and phobias related to food, selectivity in food acceptance, distrust of new foods) (Ammaniti et al. 2012).

Several studies have also investigated the quality of interactions between children diagnosed with IA and their mothers and have further evaluated the psychological profile of the mothers. Through the use of validated observational tools it was found that low dyadic reciprocity, maternal intrusiveness, high interactive conflict, negative affectivity and anhedonia characterized the affective tone, the degree of involvement and the characteristics of the interactions between mothers and their children with IA (Ammaniti et al. 2010; Chatoor, Ganiban, Hirsh, Borman-Spurrell, & Mrazek 2000; Gueron-Sela, Atzaba-Poria, Meiri, Yerushalmi 2011; Lucarelli, Cimino, D'Olimpio, & Ammaniti 2013; Stein, Woolley, & McPherson 1999). Mothers of children with IA also present a psychopathological profile, mainly characterized by depression and eating disorders (Chatoor et al. 2000; Lucarelli et al. 2013). The Italian longitudinal study that followed the natural course of a clinical sample of children diagnosed with IA, up to the age of eight years, revealed a significant association between child internalizing and externalizing problems and the psychopathological symptoms of mothers, in the absence of a psychotherapeutic treatment (Ammaniti et al. 2012). The same prospective study showed that the depressive and somatopsychic (concerns about food, body image dysfunctions, dietary restrictions) maternal psychopathology constituted a significant predictor of the interactive conflict during meals, found during infancy between the mother and the infant diagnosed with IA (Ammaniti et al. 2012). The association between depression, maternal eating disorders and a clinical condition characterized by intense and persistent food refusal of the child, with symptoms comparable to those of IA according to the DC:0–3R, by high interactive dyadic conflict between mother and child and by excessive maternal control and intrusiveness during meals was also highlighted by other studies that have investigated the development of dysfunctional eating patterns in the first three and five years of life of children of mothers with psychopathological diagnoses of eating disorders (anorexia, bulimia and eating disorders not otherwise specified) (Cooper, Whelan, Woolgar, Morrell, & Murray 2004; Stein, Woolley, & McPherson 1999). Furthermore, a recent Italian study, which compared the psychological and psychopathological profile of mothers of children diagnosed with the different diagnostic subtypes of Infantile Anorexia, Sensory Food Aversions, and Feeding Disorder associated with a Gastrointestinal Tract Disorder, showed a clinically significant condition relative to depressive symptoms and dysfunctions related to nutrition in mothers of children diagnosed with IA, in comparison with mothers of children with other specific eating disorders (Lucarelli et al. 2013), confirming previous studies on the maternal psychopathological profile.

Taken together, these studies on IA have found a disturbed pattern in relation to emotions and nutrition both in children and in their mothers, indicating that interactive dyadic conflict, maternal symptomatic features and the dysfunctional temperamental and emotional–behavioural features of children with IA are mutually implicated in the origins and persistence of this specific early-onset eating disorder.

It is also important to point out that some studies that, in these dysfunctional mother–child dyad situations, had the clinical objective of connecting the study of the eating disorder of children with early anorexia to that of family interaction processes, found decreased quality, in the responsive, supportive and structuring (of play or feeding interactions) capacities of both mothers and fathers of children with early anorexia, compared to a control group, also noting higher maternal involvement and lower paternal involvement in the relationship with their child (Atzaba-Poria et al. 2010). Furthermore, an Italian experimental study using the Lausanne Trilogue Play (LTP; Fivaz-Depeursinge & Corboz-Warnery 1999) paradigm in families of children diagnosed with Infantile Anorexia, in comparison with a control group, highlighted significant observational data concerning the difficulties of families of children with IA in finding emotional attunement, to share pleasure and emotional states co-constructed in the triadic interaction. The impact of these family dysfunctions on children with IA was also highlighted; these children, compared to the control group, show inadequate communication skills with respect to their developmental stage, highlighting low autonomy and difficulties in involvement with both parents (Lucarelli, Simonelli, & Ammaniti 2012).

The second relevant clinical condition discussed in this chapter is the Feeding Disorder associated with a Gastrointestinal Tract Disorder (Table 4.1), characterized by food refusal following a major traumatic event or repeated distressing experiences that have affected the oral-feeding system due to specific functional problems and/or invasive and/or surgical medical procedures the child underwent because of a previous organic disease, or an accidental event (for example, a domestic accident with the ingestion of toxic substances). Clinical observation has shown that these children, after the adverse oral-nutritional experiences and, persistently, after the resolution of the organic cause and the end of medical treatment, show an intense anticipatory distress during meals and considerable resistance to the intake of food in both the pre-oral and intra-oral stages and may present different levels of disorder severity with partial food refusal (for example, only towards either liquid or solid foods), or total food refusal (Benoit & Coolbear 1998; Chatoor, Ganiban, Harrison, & Hirsch 2001; Grava, Lucarelli, & Ammaniti 2014; Lucarelli et al. 2013). It is possible to observe an intense reaction of anxiety and fear in children affected by this disorder, that may appear at the mere sight of food or cooking utensils, or as meal time approaches; if forced to face the feared situation, they can sometimes develop full panic attacks. If forced to eat, these children might respond with crying, screaming, violent behaviour, refusal to open their mouths or swallow what is offered to them; sometimes they may spit out food, keep it in their mouth for a long time, or hide it to avoid having to swallow it; in some cases, food is ingested but with great distress and only after it has been blended, reduced to small pieces, or chewed for a long time (Chatoor 2009). In the most severe cases, when refusal extends to both solid and liquid foods, artificial feeding may become necessary. The reactions of children with this type of disorder are similar to those seen with Post-Traumatic Stress Disorder, with regard to the symptoms of trauma reliving, avoidance of stimuli associated with the traumatic event and decreased involvement in everyday activities (Chatoor et al. 2001). The anxiety, the anticipatory fear and the resistance towards food ingestion are associated with recurrent nightmares, night terrors with awakenings, dreams of fear of suffocation; there may be the emergence of separation anxiety, especially from the mother, and there might be an increase in the emotional dependence of the child, who might want to sleep in bed with the parents (co-sleeping); finally, the child may show irritability, social withdrawal and reduction in play activities, up to an interruption in school attendance, often in the context of a school phobia. These observations have brought about the naming of this complex clinical condition as PTED (Chatoor 2009).

In parents of children with PTED there is intense anxiety and concern: a dysfunctional and controlling parenting style during meal time characterized by very high levels of tension, conflict and poor reciprocity between adult and child that contribute to the maintenance of the child's symptoms and in some cases to their further intensification (Okada et al. 2007). The anticipatory anxiety and a greater resistance to food intake were found to be specific characteristics that significantly differentiate children with this type of disorder in a clinical sample that had experienced oral-feeding adverse events originating from a severe gastro-oesophageal reflux disease in their first three years of life, compared with children who had IA (Chatoor et al. 2001; Lucarelli et al. 2013). A finding that emerged from the study of mother–infant feeding interactions in the context of PTED and that may be particularly interesting and significant in guiding therapeutic interventions, relates to significant associations, in mothers and children with PTED, between dyadic affective states and all dysfunctional dimensions of food resistance. In particular, the more food interactions are characterized by conflicting aspects and negative affective states, the more the child's resistance to food increases. Therefore, the feeding interactive patterns are characterized by aspects of dysfunctionality both in maternal behaviour and in that of the child, and the history of adverse traumatic oral-feeding events sits at the origin of a problematic condition that is reflected both at an individual and relational level (Grava et al. 2014; Lucarelli et al. 2013).

Research in this field has also highlighted meal-time father–child dyadic interactions characterized by low dyadic reciprocity and a lack of sharing of positive affect: like mothers, fathers may also have difficulties in supporting the self-regulating abilities of the child (Grava et al. 2014). Furthermore, if the mothers of these children, differently from those of children with IA, do not present more specific psychopathological conditions such as depression and eating disorders, they show clinically significant anxiety (Lucarelli et al. 2013). The same clinical study, investigating the emotion regulation of children with previous medical and pathological history of gastro-oesophageal reflux, highlighted a clinically significant condition in the regulation of aggression, mainly characterized by irritability, temper tantrums, excessive crying, frustration, excessive dependence and demands for attention. Of note, an assessment of these children's temperament also showed clinically significant scores in "inhibition to novelty" (Lucarelli et al. 2013). Considering the history of traumatic oral-feeding experiences of these children, it is plausible that this emotional dysregulation and temperamental inhibition could contribute to further stabilize the eating disorder. Other clinically significant variables that emerged were the anxious symptomatology of mothers and the fathers' difficulties in compensating for the problematic outcomes in a context of less-than-optimal interactions with the child. This may all compromise the ability of parents to contain and moderate the impact of the traumatic feeding experience on the child's emotion regulation and adaptive behaviour. The role of the family therefore emerges as an important element in determining both the development and the course of the pathology and may represent either a risk factor or a protective factor, in relation to the onset of the symptomatology and its level of severity (Grava et al. 2014).

3. Infantile Anorexia and Post-Traumatic Eating Disorder: parent–child interactions and clinical intervention

The complex diagnostic process is a fundamental step, not just to reach a clearer understanding of the clinical condition, but also and most of all to define the best clinical treatment strategy for each specific type of disorder.

In Infantile Anorexia, given the high interactive conflict between mother and child and the clinical manifestations in emotion and psychosomatic regulation of both children and their mothers, the therapeutic approach should have a double focus both on the child and on the parents. Parent–child psychotherapy and family-oriented relational–systemic interventions are particularly appropriate when the behavioural problems of the infant disorder, the dysfunctional profiles of the parents' personalities and the relational context compromise the communicative skills and the parental functions of adequate support to the child's developmental processes (Fivaz-Depeursinge 2008; Fivaz-Depeursinge & Corboz-Warnery 1999).

As previously described, the use of video-feedback, applied to the specific context of mother–child feeding interactions, represents the possibility of promoting and increasing the parents' awareness of their interactions with their child and their ability to reflect on their own states of mind and those of their child, initially with particular reference to the problematic feeding experience they are going through with their child.

In the specific clinical context of IA, in which the disorder is associated with poor child growth, parental hyper-vigilance is often present in relation to the somatic components (weight of the child, quantity and types of food consumed, intense concerns focused on food refusal). These dynamics can limit the parent's abilities – especially those of the mother in her function as primary caregiver at meal-time – to be responsive to the child's attempts to communicate with the parent and to express mental states and intentions in the relationship.

During the first psychological assessment visit, carried out on the GP's recommendation for a problem of poor growth (with no apparent organic cause) of Francesca, who is three years old, her mother very carefully takes a booklet out of her bag; she immediately says that she also showed it to the GP. In this booklet, Ms M. every night, without fail – she comments – writes how much and what Francesca eats and calculates the nutrients ingested, with the help of a table she found on the Internet. Based on this calculation, Ms M. explains, she decides the integration of nutrients that she will put in the bottle of milk she will give to her daughter when she is about to fall asleep.

This is the only way, according to her, that her child accepts eating. The video-recorded observation of a meal with Francesca and Ms M., proposed by the psychologist, highlights the characteristics of the eating behaviour of the child who shows neither interest nor initiative towards food, but seems completely absorbed by the activity of drawing by changing deftly, but in a sudden and repetitive way, the use of many coloured markers that she takes out of a bag; the mother, commenting several times "you can't live on milk alone" offers small meatballs (food that the child occasionally likes), but she seems passively resigned to an expectation of refusal by her daughter who, keeping her head down on the drawing, stubbornly repeats "no Mom, I don't want it". Within the treatment programme, a suggestion is made to the mother to work on meal-time mother–child interactions, motivated by the need to establish a diet that is suitable for the child's age and by the importance of being able to overcome the anomalies in the eating behaviour of Francesca, who should have already achieved an internal regulation of hunger/satiety and the ability to eat by herself. Gradually a change is suggested in the structure of the meal, the mother will no longer spoon-feed the child, but Francesca will have an active role and will be able to make decisions, even to eat little during one meal and more during the next one, negotiating with her mother a minimum amount of food until she feels full; adequate nutritional advice will help the mother to eliminate the evening milk bottle and the ritual calculation of nutrients ingested by the child. After a few months, Francesca's IA improves significantly, the amount of food she eats is still limited, but the use of milk bottles is now completely replaced by meals at the table, in the presence of her father as well. Francesca's mother begins a psychotherapy, after "realizing", she says, "that like her daughter she too needs to learn to feel when she is hungry". From adolescence, Ms M. has suffered from a restrictive anorexic disorder; she keeps her eating in check, and almost always "skips lunch" because, she says, "she is too stressed and busy to think about eating". The elaboration of the interactive conflict with Francesca during meals has triggered a profound and positive journey of change for Ms M.

Starting from the phase of feedback of the diagnostic process to parents, the video-feedback clinical intervention shifts the attentional focus of parents from concerns about nutrition and the somatic symptoms to the quality of emotional communication with their child. This allows, as was highlighted by Fivaz-Depeursinge (2008), a shift from a negative semiotics, in which attention is focused on dysfunctional and pathological aspects of the child and of the relationship, to a positive semiotics that focuses on the child's abilities and resources and those of the child's context of significant relationships. Furthermore, the use of video-feedback can produce very important results in relation to the child's active role – from the first months of life – in the co-construction of the interactive patterns that define the environment which in turn affects the child's development, with significant clinical implications, such as negotiating with the child the possibility of contributing to change in therapy.

Video-feedback can prove useful in the phases of feedback of the diagnostic process and of therapeutic proposal, and in clinical interventions associated with psychotherapeutic sessions aimed at the parent and/or the parental couple (Corboz-Warnery 2014). In this direction, the guided observation of the "dysfunctional" interactive patterns constitutes a clinical intervention strategy to promote insightfulness and the ability to reflect on the current relationship with the child, that is, the ability of parents of children in treatment to see the problematic behaviour from the latter's point of view and at the same time to be able to empathically understand the implicit motivations of the children's problematic behaviour (Koren-Karie, Oppenheim, & Goldsmith 2010; Sameroff, McDonough, & Rosenblum 2004).

Video-feedback enables parents to experience a real-time interaction and then observe it, experimenting with it again after some time; interactions can be slowed down and it is possible to carefully examine the different levels of communication and affect – verbal, non-verbal, relating to tone, expressions and gazes – proving what a valuable tool for change it can be (Corboz-Warnery 2014).

Giorgia is 11 months of age when her mother requests a GP visit because the child vomits during meals; the problem started a few months before with the introduction of the first baby foods. The episodes of "vomiting" do not seem to occur if the child is fed with the bottle. Ms C. thinks that the child has a "stomach problem" that causes the vomiting; she also thinks she was wrong to stop breastfeeding, as the child had not accepted this change. She describes Giorgia as a "stubborn", "bossy" child, "she wants to touch everything", "we must control everything she does". The father claims that the child "is like him who has always been thin", even when he was little he didn't want to eat. He emphasizes the aspects of "normality" of Giorgia, she is cheerful, she is lively, "she is a normal child". The GP evaluation and the medical examinations exclude an organic aetiology, noting, however, the poor growth of the child and her being underweight. Psychological counselling is provided, in which an observation of the mother–child feeding interaction is suggested. Ms C. wants to put Giorgia in a high chair, and comments "otherwise I can't get her to eat, she is always on the move, she never stops", and while the child tries to grab the spoon, Ms C. quickly moves the plate outside her daughter's reach, and tries to spoon-feed the girl who refuses, Ms C. mechanically gives her a toy, without showing any pleasure and enthusiasm, while at the same time she energetically shoves the spoon into the child's mouth, several episodes are repeated one after the other, the child shuts her mouth, cries loudly, Ms C. with one hand covers the child's eyes while pressing on her cheeks she forces her to open her mouth brusquely forcing feeding, the child regurgitates the soup, she cries so intensely and is so distressed that she only calms down 20 minutes later. The video-feedback session that followed enabled Ms C. to re-experience the interactive conflict and the intense emotional distress in a non-judgmental, supportive context of reflection about the "battlefield" between her and her daughter; Ms C. was helped to recognize, focusing on the sequence filmed at the beginning of the meal, the signs of autonomy of Giorgia, entirely appropriate for her age and the importance of sharing with the child her new and different psychological rhythms towards autonomous feeding. Giorgia's father comments: "now that I see what happens I realize, maybe I'm wrong to go to another room, but I can't hear the child crying and screaming that way!" The feedback of the video-feedback session activated cooperation dynamics in the parental couple, which rapidly led to experimenting with the father's supportive sharing of the child's meal-times. Longer were the times of elaboration of the unresolved mourning of Giorgia's mother who, as her affective story showed, had traumatically lost her mother when she was three due to an accident. The early experience of affective loss made it difficult for Ms C. to internalize effective parental models to face her current maternal role, especially with reference to the psychodynamic processes involved in her daughter's dependence and autonomy. During the course of the treatment, supporting the development of the girl's autonomy patterns, which the father contributed towards, was found to be effective, as this facilitated the re-establishment of communicative exchanges and the child herself can offer her mother, now more receptive, a clearer procedural model to satisfy her physiological and emotional needs, which had previously been compromised by dysfunctional interactive adjustments.

Improving the quality of interactions between child and parents can often quickly reduce the difficulties in child emotion regulation, increasing the satisfaction that both parent and children get from their interactions and promoting resources and a more positive context to address more complex problems and dysfunctions in the family unit.

It is important to point out that an intervention that addresses the observable interactive behaviours does not exclude, but rather promotes care focused on the internal experience of the parents and on the level of the parental mental representations that guide and support the quality of the actual interactive behaviours. The intrapsychic representational system and the interpersonal behavioural system involved in the parent–child relationships can in fact be considered as interconnected and the changes that occur in one system affect the other in a reciprocal manner (Stern 2004).

In summary, parent–child psychotherapy aims to go beyond the problematic behaviour of the child through a reformulation of negative and distorted representations and offering a complex view of the child with limits and resources and favouring reflective parental function, that is, a way of thinking of the child as a separate person with feelings, needs, desires and personal motivations.

Although many of the clinical reflections presented and many of the scientific literature references reported could also be applied to interventions aimed at eating disorders associated with adverse organic experiences in the child's history, the specific clinical aspects of PTED need to be highlighted. In particular, as previously evidenced in this chapter, the anticipatory anxiety and the emotional dysregulation of the child as reactions to adverse oral-feeding experiences, indicate that the therapeutic approach should be based on a multidisciplinary intervention. In cases of malnutrition and/or growth difficulties that compromise the overall development of the child, intensive care and often the work of a multidisciplinary team are necessary, as medical–nutritional interventions may be necessary, as well as, in some cases, rehabilitation interventions aimed at the child's eating functions, and specialized psychotherapeutic treatments. In particular, in the presence of previous medical and/or surgical events addressing oral/feeding issues, it may be necessary to restore normal nutrition, to use rehabilitation techniques and desensitization of traumatic oral-feeding outcomes, together with the provision of psychological support to parents.

The main challenge for children with PTED is to resolve the intense fear of food associated with their traumatic experience. In this specific area of intervention, in the existing scientific literature, there are some interesting clinical contributions that have shown the effectiveness of desensitization treatments, in the most serious cases in association with child oral-feeding function rehabilitation techniques, performed in a psychodynamic and relational therapeutic context that involves the child's family in multidisciplinary outpatient and residential clinical services for diagnosis and treatment, specialized in dealing with this particular type of child eating disorder (Benoit, Coolbear 1998; Chatoor 2009; Dunitz-Scheer et al. 2011). In these clinical contexts, the use of video-feedback and psychological support for parents is essential, often to prevent dysfunctional parent–child interactive modalities that may become established, such as feeding children while they sleep, when the children accept liquid foods, or trying to feed the child at any time of the day.

As previously noted, studies on children who had distressing experiences affecting their oral-feeding system and who developed a PTED found a comorbidity between this disorder and anxiety disorders. In particular, the history of older children often reveals that they suffered from clinically significant anxiety before the onset of the PTED, highlighting a pre-existing psychological vulnerability of the child and of the family affective ties, especially in relation to a developmental conflict involving separation anxiety (Chatoor 1996, 2009). The distressing oral-feeding event would therefore seem to increase the child's anxiety and crystallize anxiety around the fear of food and suffocation. Once this clinical condition of "terror of food" has become established, no degree of reasoning seems able to convince these children not to be worried and that they will not have problems swallowing food; the child may quickly lose weight. The child's anxiety spreads, involving other life areas: difficulties in falling asleep, in concentrating, school phobia, social withdrawal behaviour.

Tiziana is a three-and-a-half year old girl with a history of oesophageal atresia. A year ago she underwent a resolutive surgical intervention for her organic-functional pathology, the clinical course was optimal, and Tiziana's nutrition should have evolved according to normal and regular patterns. It became instead necessary to start a psychological evaluation due to the very high level of tension of Ms S., mother of Tiziana, and to the dysfunctional eating pattern of the child. Ms S. reports, in fact, that the child ingests exclusively, but with difficulty, blended food, she refuses any solid food, and has recently started refusing liquids as well. Because of these problems, Tiziana's mother has decided not to let Tiziana attend nursery school, while she took a leave of absence from work in order to be able to dedicate herself completely to her child. As for Tiziana, in these first years of her life, she has always had to deal with separation anxiety when her mother had to be away from her, even during sleep; every night, now, the child sleeps in her mother's bed; Tiziana's father sleeps in another room. The video-recorded observation at meal-times shows Tiziana's intense anticipatory anxiety at the mere sight of the dish with the blended food, she cries immediately and intensely; the meal is totally controlled by her mother who, in between useless attempts to calm the child, force-feeds the girl with a spoon, while Tiziana occasionally swallows the food offered, crying continuously, bringing her hand up to cover her mouth, tightly closing her lips, and occasionally swallowing the food, completely exhausted. The following video-feedback session focuses on feedback with the aim of helping the mother understand the symptoms of terror of food that have become organized in the child and the need to modify the controlling behaviour of the mother, which, although brought about by her intense concern, not only has no effect if the child does not cooperate, but is also the cause of an increase in symptoms. In the treatment plan, the nutritionist recommends to Ms S. a list of different soft foods that the child can swallow easily; parents are advised to encourage the child to eat alone, starting with small amounts of food, and to eat some of the same foods the child has, so as to offer her a positive and reassuring model. During the psychologist's clinical interview with both parents, Tiziana's mother seems to speak without taking a breath, as she comments that "hospital is – for her – like a second home"; she talks about the long illness of her father, affected by severe cardiopathy, the numerous admissions to hospital since she was eight years old until she was 17, when her father died, after spending several years bedridden. She talks in great detail about her active role in her father's medical care, and how much time she spent in his company to help him feel less alone. She talks about the bitter conflict with her mother, about the strong misunderstandings between them, which led to their relationship breaking up some years before. Ms S. expresses her intense pain for her mother's absence at the time of the birth of her baby, as her mother had not accepted her choice of partner and her marriage, for reasons that she still cannot understand. Tiziana's medical diagnosis, formulated a few months after birth and following difficulties in breastfeeding due to the girl's intense and continuous regurgitations, amplified a pre-existing anxiety, creating, in the mother, a continuous state of alarm about her daughter's health and resulting in an extremely controlling parenting style from which the husband says he feels "excluded" and which has led him to increasingly retreat into a passive role of "defeat". Clinical work carried out in parallel with a double focus on the parental couple and on the feeding interactions with the child showed a gradual improvement in Tiziana's PTED. The father has changed his work shifts and in the evening is always present at meal-time with his daughter; after a few months, Tiziana is able to eat different foods, with a reduced variety, but of different consistency, and above all, her anticipatory anxiety towards food has decreased significantly. The video-feedback sessions, carried out during follow-up sessions, showed the father as gradually more able to support the child's emotion regulation, how Tiziana's mother gradually reduced her intrusive and anticipatory behaviours, bringing greater vitality in the interaction, and how the family shows greater cohesion that will help them reinforce the co-parental alliance. The inclusion of the father within the relationship between the mother and the child, at meal- and sleep-times, activated a process of affective differentiation with a positive impact on Tiziana's separation anxiety problem and the experimentation of new and age-appropriate developmental models, such as having her own room to sleep by herself and beginning to attend nursery school. The therapeutic process, which dealt with the problems of Tiziana and her family in its entirety, ensured that the significantly compromised development of the child could be restored.

Numerous intervention programmes have confirmed childhood as a critical and particularly sensitive period for early interventions that could have very significant positive outcomes, such as the reduction of maladaptive behaviours, the increase of attachment behaviours and the improvement of emotion and affect regulation strategies. Experimental research on and clinical experiences with early-onset eating disorders have confirmed that many "symptoms" of the relevant clinical conditions, examined in this chapter, are transactional and dependent on the interpersonal context of family relationships and emphasize the need for timely interventions focused on the *here* and *now* and aimed at parent–child interactions and the parental couple. Specifically, the Mindful Emotion Regulation approach proposed by the authors aims to support parents in understanding the child's behaviour, suspending judgement and welcoming an attribution of meaning based on emotional states, ultimately thinking about it more in terms of the child's internal experience rather than the child's behaviour; at the same time parents are encouraged to pay attention to the child's internal experience, which is progressively recognized as separate from them.

Highlights

- This chapter offered a detailed description of the clinical evaluation and of two relevant clinical conditions, Infantile Anorexia (AI) and Post-Traumatic Feeding Disorder (PTFD), highlighting how the approach of choice for clinical evaluation and treatment should have a double focus on both the child and the parents.

- In parents of children with PTFD, a dysfunctional and controlling parenting style is observed at meal-time, characterized by very high levels of tension, conflict and poor reciprocity between adult and child. AI presents high interactive conflict between the caregiver and the child.
- Clinical intervention through video-feedback, applied to the specific context of caregiver–child food interactions, represents today the possibility of promoting and increasing the awareness of parents in relation to their interactions with their child, and their ability to reflect on each other's mental states.
- Video-feedback allows parents to experience a feeding interaction in real time and then to observe it, experimenting with it again after some time; interactions can be slowed down and it is possible to deeply analyse their different communicative and affective levels – verbal, non-verbal, relating to tone, expressions and looks, proving to be a valuable tool for change.
- Video-feedback can find applications in the feedback phase of the diagnostic process and therapeutic proposal, and in clinical interventions in association with psychotherapeutic sessions aimed at the parent and/or the parental couple.
- The guided observation of the "dysfunctional" interactive patterns constitutes a clinical intervention strategy to promote insightfulness and the ability to reflect on the current relationship with the child, that is, the ability of the parents of the children being treated to be able to see the problematic behaviour from their child's point of view and at the same time to be able to empathically understand the implicit motivations of their child's problematic behaviour.

Notes

1 With Karen Kaye's (1982) definition of *scaffolding*, intended as a parental action towards young infants, the interactive–cognitive approach shines a light on the supportive adult function of creating *frames*, that is micro-structures tailored around the infant. For example, the continuity of maternal gaze during early feeding, which represents an integrating background for the new-born's experience, or when parents, interpreting the infant's intentions, perform actions the infant seemed intent on achieving, offering a modelling framework, and then waiting for the infant to try and imitate them, to provide meaning to these actions in a shared social context.

2 The Diagnostic Classification of Mental Health and Developmental Disorder of Infancy and Early Childhood – DC:0–3R (Zero-To-Three 2005), now in its first revision, refers to multiaxial factors that can contribute to children's difficulties; the suggested diagnostic categories are of both a descriptive, that is to say they indicate a set of symptoms and behaviours of children and parents, and an etiological kind, that is they indicate individual characteristics of the parent, the child and their relationship, as causal sources of the disorder, especially thanks to the innovative

introduction of Axis II for the classification of the quality of the parent–child relationship. Axis II, which represents one of the main strengths of this diagnostic system, identifies the understanding of the quality of the parent–child relationship as an essential part of the clinical formulation and of any treatment programme in childhood. This approach represents an important guarantee to safeguard the complexity of the clinical evaluation and to be able to take into account the intertwining of individual and relational variables that may be associated with a functional developmental disorder, such as eating disorders in childhood. In accordance with the "Research Diagnostic Criteria – Preschool Age" of the American Academy of Child and Adolescent Psychiatry (Task Force on Research Diagnostic Criteria: Infancy and Preschool 2003), the DC:0–3R defines different diagnostic subtypes of eating disorders in preschool age. These disorders differ in terms of developmental period and manifestations at onset, their symptomatic configuration, their clinical course and their level of severity.

3 Sensory Food Aversions in infancy, characterized by the selective refusal of foods due to their sensorial characteristics and by the difficulty in trying new ones, generally constitute non-severe feeding and eating developmental psychopathological conditions. Psychological counselling to help parents provide adequate support to the emotional state of the child with sensory aversions is necessary to prevent certain problematic outcomes of food selectivity that have been associated with social phobia, generalized anxiety, obsessive–compulsive symptoms and academic difficulties (Lucarelli et al. 2013; Nicholls and Jaffa 2007).

Chapter 5

Food refusal in preschool-age children

Elena Trombini and Giancarlo Trombini

1. Problems with eating and emotion regulation in preschool age

Studies on eating disorders in preschool age underline the importance of assessing the individual characteristics of the child and his relationships within the family, which can be at the origin of a difficult correspondence between the self-regulatory and behavioural styles of the child and the expectations of the adults, influenced in turn by their past experiences with their caregivers. Literature has also highlighted that childhood eating disorders tend to persist, representing risk factors for the development of growth disorders, behavioural problems and personality disorders (Benoit 1996; Bryant-Waugh, Markham, Kreipe, & Walsh 2010; Chatoor 1996; Lebovici, Diatkine, & Soulé 1990; Lucarelli 2001). This continuity between developmental and adult psychopathology is fully reflected in the latest revision of the DSM-5 (APA 2013), in which eating disorders are included in a single section called "Feeding and Eating Disorders".

Clinical approaches therefore carefully focus on the quality of the adult/child relationship and are oriented towards the early identification and intervention on dysfunctional relationships with parental figures.

In clinical–diagnostic categories (DSM-5, PDM-2), eating disorders that can be seen as "symptoms of psychosomatic protest" become particularly important (Trombini 1994; Trombini 2002, 2010, 2011; Trombini & Trombini 2006, 2007): at the origin of these disorders there is a frustration, by the adult, of the motivation, in children, to do things by themselves, in relation to food and eating. In fact, under normal conditions, the establishment of eating habits, and subsequently of those related to hygiene, which lead to behaviours highly appreciated and expected by the adult, should not be considered the result of imposed learning, but should instead be considered intimately connected with the motivation to do things by oneself, which is expressed in the context of a harmonious shared life. Requests to do things by oneself attest on the one hand an awareness of the anchoring of the undertaken activity to the Self and on the other also the initial exercise of one's will: a sense of being, existing and being the cause of one's own actions. In this sense, the Self as an anchoring point for one's own actions is placed in good succession with a primary nuclear Self, organized around bodily experiences, endowed with creative and productive potential and which provides a meaning to life (Arfelli Galli 1995; Lang & Rivolta 2015; Molinari & Lappi 1994).

The request to do by oneself reaches its climax in the second and third year of life. A characteristic of this period is the consolidation of neuromuscular mastery associated with the acquisition of walking that facilitates exploration and promotes further activities. Therefore, there is an increasing refinement of the conduct supported by the motivation to do things by oneself which is expressed as a natural evolution of the tendency to develop an active relationship with the environment (Stern, 1989, 1992; Trevarthen 1990, 1998).

Klamma, as early as in 1957, provided empirical evidence for the children's desire to do by themselves with objects of their daily environment (which can be observed around the age of two), definable as a lively request to do things by themselves associated with a refusal of the adult's offer of help. This conduct is not aimed at achieving a certain level of performance, but simply at the pleasure of "doing things independently". In fact, at the first sign of difficulties in performing a given task, children desist in their intentions and ask for the help they had previously refused.[1] This can be seen at least up to the age of four. These are behaviours that, even though not yet motivated by obtaining a successful result, require awareness of the anchoring of the undertaken activities to the Self: a sense of being, as underlined by Vallino and Macciò (2004), and of being the cause of the one's own actions.

Giancarlo Trombini was the first to point out (1969) that, in order to be translated into behaviour, the motivation to do things by oneself requires an adequate stimulus, which, in relation to food and eating, is the configuration of food as something pleasing to put inside oneself and, in relation to evacuation, as something to be eliminated. Specifically, clinical investigations have shown that this motivation appears in the second year for eating conduct and in the third for defecation and urination (Baldaro & Trombini 1989; Baldaro, Trombini, & Trombini 1994; Baldaro 2002; Canestrari & Trombini 1975; Trombini 2002, 2008, 2010; Trombini 1969, 1970).

Finally, it should be noted that in the process of development, its original tendency (Lichtenberg 1995), as a motivation to do by oneself, can be made conflicting or favoured by the family environment, which not only stimulates it, but enables it, through previous satisfactory attachment experiences (Battacchi & Giovanelli 1988). When children can consider themselves members who enjoy the same respect as other family members, a harmonious shared life is facilitated in which enacting behaviours supported by the motivation to do by oneself can be in agreement both with the feeling of "being an I", but also with that of being part of a family "Us". Conversely, the impossibility of inserting oneself without friction in the reality of the order of family life, due to adult coercive interventions, can bring about a painful sense of isolation in the child. Protest behaviours can therefore be triggered (such as not wanting to eat, vomiting, not wanting to defecate, wetting the bed) with which children signal the inadequacy of those looking after them and try to regain the lost autonomy.

2. The psychotherapeutic intervention

Problems inherent to the eating behaviour of preschool-aged children are particularly frequent and require careful observation by clinicians to diagnose and distinguish transitory forms from pathological conditions, in order to propose targeted interventions able to free the child and parents from the "suffering imprisoned in the symptom" (Vallino 2009).

By listening to mothers and fathers who describe in detail, often with distressing lucidity, how much and how their children do not eat, vomit, spit, oppose spoon-feeding and solid foods, one is immersed in an emotional climate in which the concreteness of the eating problem takes on such dimensions as to saturate the reflective abilities of the adult (Trombini 2010). Therefore, staying with the suffering of parents and children with eating problems at an early age, that is, when communication does not mainly take place through the verbal channel, and proposing a support intervention are very complex and involving tasks.

In this regard, it should be underlined that nowadays the vision of child psychotherapy has changed. In fact, although differences remain in the various authors' paradigms and approaches to the clinical work in developmental age, recent decades have seen the theoretical landscape and the focus of evaluation and intervention shift towards the child–parent relationship, believing seeing children together with their family to be essential (Busato Barbaglio & Mondello 2011; Lanyado & Horne 2003; Neri & Latmiral 2004; Sameroff, DcDonough, & Rosenblum 2004; Trombini, De Pascalis, & Neri 2015; Tsiantis, Boethious, Hallerfors, Horne, & Tischler 2002; Vallino 2007; Vallino & Macciò 2011).

Literature has widely emphasized the primary role that affects, parent–child emotional attunement, and interpersonal relationships have in the psychic development of the individual. In this regard, de Campora and Zavattini (2011, 2015) summarize how in current psychoanalytic models there is the idea of a closer relationship between the profile of the internal world and the real relationships, making the interpersonal dimension the scenario on which to base more specifically intrapsychic aspects. In this context, intersubjectivity can be thought of as a basic motivational system (Stern 2005) that guides the child from his first experiences (Riva Crugnola 2007). A child "in relation" emerges (de Campora & Zavattini, 2011), who is influenced and in turn influences his surrounding environment. The study of preverbal relationships also shows that, as Vallino and Macciò (2012) highlighted, the child's mind becomes accessible to the observer, in its affective and cognitive complexity, only in the "here and now" of the participation of the parents who share the child's everyday life.

The history of child psychotherapy teaches us that parents have long been left out of the therapist's room (Algini 2007). It was a defensive strategy both to quickly establish intimacy with the child and to avoid intense emotional involvement with the family members' tormented feelings. Nowadays, however, as stated by Dina Vallino (2011), leading parents back to rediscovering their child as a person is a prerequisite for being able to explore the children's creativity and take care of their inhibitions, allowing parents to be helped in becoming the "experts" they potentially are. The child disorder associated with the family crisis requires reference models equally centred on the intrapsychic relationship and on the interpersonal relationship, like what happens in real everyday life between parents and children.

The "Participated Consultation" (PC) methodology with children and parents proposed by Dina Vallino (2009) enables the reactivation of the mental bond between family members. Through this methodology, the author not only provides valuable indications regarding early preventive intervention, but she also outlines a vision of child psychoanalysis that "puts children at the centre of their world", in which parents are an essential part.[2] Participated Consultation is in fact able to help parents to (re)discover their children who, since infancy, "wave their psychic existence" (Vallino & Macciò 2004), giving parents back the responsibility of their own competence on their children.

It is within this frame of reference that "Focal Play-Therapy" (FPT) is presented as a specific preventive–therapeutic intervention approach that enables one to deal with eating disorders in preschool age with parents and children, restarting a transformative process capable of returning children to the care of their parents, who, at the same time, can claim back their personal parental skills. This is facilitated by the proposed methodology, as it enables one to pay attention to what happens in the *here and now*, offering an opportunity to show parents "how to be together" in play, observing and listening to the child.

3. Focal Play-Therapy with children and their parents: theory and technique

In the context of psychoanalytically oriented interventions, Focal Play-Therapy (FPT) was expressly designed by Giancarlo Trombini (1969; 1994) as a *specific methodology* for preschoolers with *eating and evacuation disorders*, interpretable as symptoms of *psychosomatic protest*. FPT was later adopted and introduced in the diagnostic–therapeutic process extended to parents (Trombini & Trombini 2006; 2007; Trombini 2008, 2010, 2011; Trombini, De Pascalis, & Neri 2015), according to the methodology of Dina Vallino's Participated Consultation (PC) (Vallino, 2002a, 2002b, 2007, 2009). FPT thus places itself in the current clinical context, which pays increasing attention to the narrative dimension of the young patients in their family contexts.

FPT enables one to highlight characteristics of autonomy in the relationship with food and with evacuative contents. In fact, it is based on an organized starting point that allows children to express their motivation to do things by themselves in a self-regulated conduct and which, at the same time, develops the alliance with the parents and the integration of the family group. It therefore offers a new reference system, so as to encourage in children behaviours that are appropriate to their real developmental needs.

FPT will first be presented in its essential details (Trombini 2010). The focus will then be shifted to the peculiar characteristics of the methodology used in the context of PC (with children and parents), highlighting the transformative potential for the child's suffering within the family context.

The therapist, after having established a warm and friendly contact with the child, proposes a temporal sequence in which the protagonist is a playdough puppet (usually referred to as Lewie) which, guided by the therapist, performs the basic physiological functions seen in childhood (feeding, evacuation). The therapist's voice is lent to the puppet, making it speak and act towards the request and introduction of foods made of playdough (little meatballs) the flavour of which the puppet shows appreciation for. The desire to urinate and defecate in the potty or in the toilet, built there and then with playdough, is then manifested, followed by exclamations of relief and well-being, while the playdough faeces fall into the toilet.

I further explain the proposal of the FPT sequence, with reference to Figures 5.1, 5.2 and 5.3 which illustrate it.

1   The therapists propose making a puppet (which they themselves build), to which they offer food (meatballs, candies …) made with pieces of playdough, which, one by one, they place on the mouth of the puppet, while exclaiming "what a nice smell, I'm so hungry!" (Figure 5.1).
2   After personally imitating a chewing movement, they also exclaim: "Oh, how yummy!" They then slide the pieces of food along the body of the puppet, fixing them on its belly (Figure 5.2).
3   Finally they add "What a big belly I have … I am so full, I need to poo … and pee … I'm going to do both". Therapists then build a potty/toilet on which they place the puppet from which they detach the pieces of playdough (food that has now become faeces) fixed to its belly, letting them fall into the potty/toilet: "Pluf, Pluf, oh! Much better. My tummy is empty: I did so much poop! Now I also need to pee … I will (Psss, Psss, Psss) … now I can go play … eat again … go to bed" (Figure 5.3).

Therapists then ask the children if they want food to be prepared again for the puppet. If the child accepts, the entire sequence is repeated, allowing the child to intervene personally, for example by suggesting variations in the foods (spaghetti, pizza) and in their preparation (pots, oven).

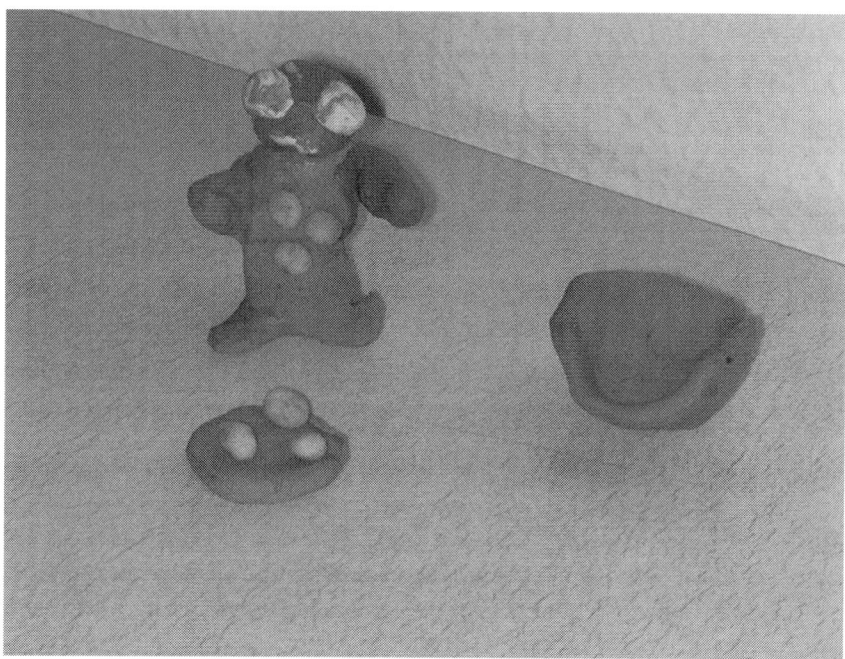

Figure 5.1 Gigetto is looking at the delicious food he would like to eat: those little pieces, brought to the mouth at first, then slip in his tummy.

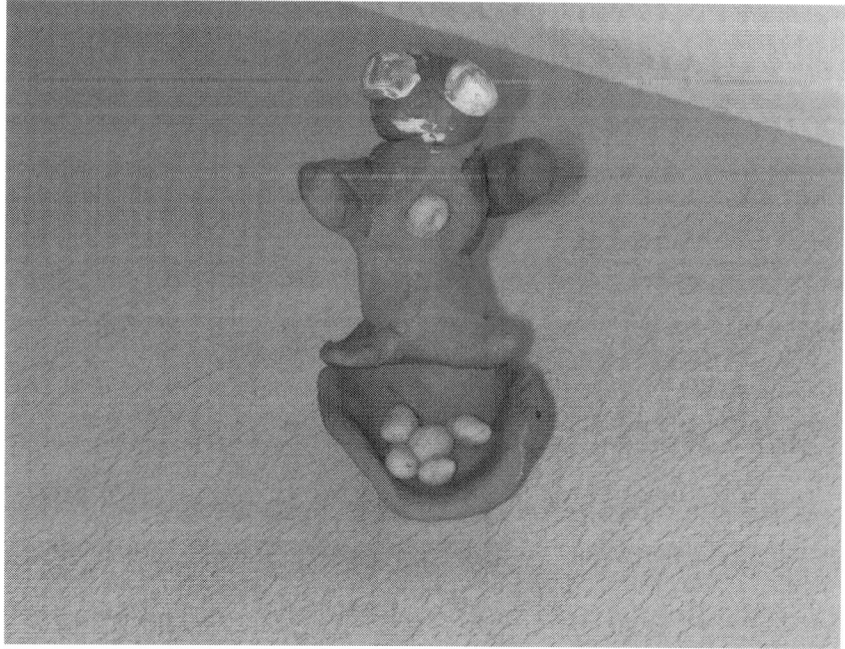

Figure 5.2 Gigetto is feeling full and he would like to evacuate. Those little pieces of food become stools, and they are now ready to fall into the toilet.

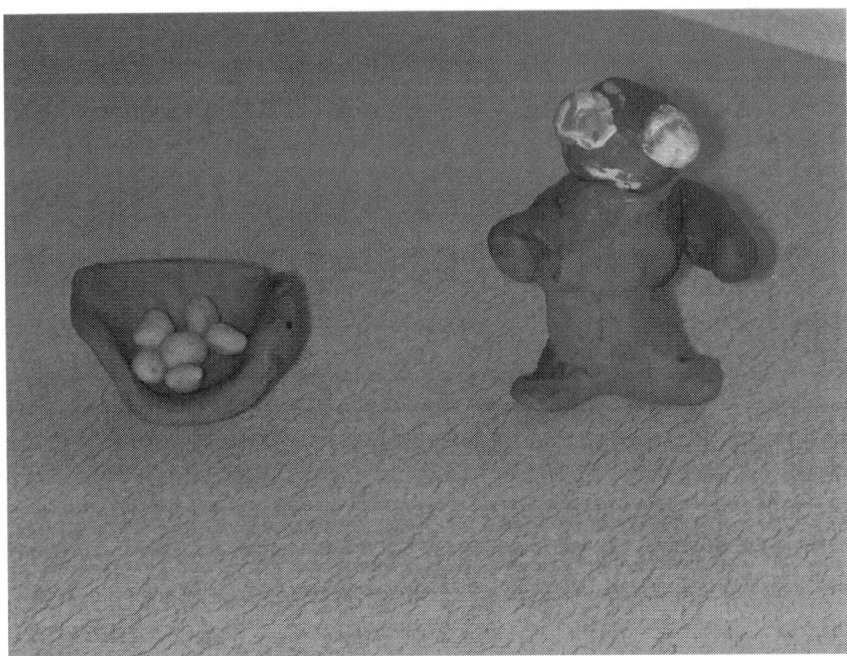

Figure 5.3 After Gigetto has eaten and evacuated, he is free to play, eat again, and go to sleep.

The therapists move in a reference system that shows the natural phenomenical qualities of foods and bodily contents, respectively as "something pleasing to put inside oneself" and as "something to be eliminated". They seek to restore the "value" of foods and bodily contents by proposing direct contact with them through the choice of foods, their preparation, the decision to eat them, the need to evacuate and the desire to do it in the place that is appropriate for shared family life.

They clarify their meaning by integrating eating and evacuation as part of a single process. In this way, food and evacuative contents are clearly configured in their natural aspect. The focus is on the phenomenical qualities of these stimuli, so that children, driven by their motivation to do things by themselves, feel attracted towards establishing direct and independent contact with them. The FPT sequence offers children a different reference system from that experienced in the family when adults interfere with their self-regulation processes, such as those related to eating and to sphincter control (Metzger 2000). In fact, the adult should offer suggestions leaving the child free to follow them. Otherwise, in the context of nutrition, food could be experienced as "something to be refused" and, if necessary, to be vomited, while with regard to evacuation, bodily contents may be configured as "something to give or to retain", in response to the impositions and demands of the adult.

Subsequently, after presenting the FPT sequence, therapists gradually withdraw into the background, allowing children to externalize and project their psychic contents onto the game, in particular those of an aggressive nature: in this way they become game themes that may find, as the therapeutic intervention proceeds, a gradual non-conflictual resolution. Therapists intervene, when appropriate, with comments expressed in a simple way and only referring to what takes place in the events of the game, or with suggestions on possible alternative solutions to the events being played out. Clinical experiences and investigations conducted in this regard (Trombini & Trombini 2006; 2007; Trombini 2010; 2011; Trombini, De Pascalis, & Neri 2015) highlight that, when an active collaboration of the child is established, associated with the spontaneous and complete execution of the feeding–evacuation sequence, normalization of feeding and evacuation in the family environment can be seen.

For the first ten cases treated with FPT (Trombini, 1969), non-spontaneous remission was indicated by the nature itself of the results. These consisted in the evident coincidence of the appearance, during treatment, of an active collaboration of the child associated on the one hand with the complete execution of the feeding–evacuation sequence and on the other with the control of feeding and evacuation in the family atmosphere.

The subsequent clinical experience of FPT implemented in the context of Participated Consultation (Trombini et al. 2015) confirmed that when such active collaboration of the child is established over the course of play-therapy and is associated with the spontaneous execution of the feeding–evacuation sequence, harmony emerges in family life, with a resolution of protest symptoms.

Focal Play-Therapy in the context of Participated Consultation allows parents to take part in their child's play and to grasp the real interests expressed in it, their child's desires, fears and angers.

In line with the model proposed by Vallino, the structure of the sessions consists of alternating play sessions with the child and parents and sessions with only the parental couple. It should be noted, however, that FPT, in this wider context, remains a psychotherapy only aimed at the child and is not a family therapy or a parental therapy. Rather, as Vallino points out, it becomes a unique opportunity for the child to "talk" about himself with the parents there, and for the latter to talk to him. It follows that for parents, in greater contact with the child, it is a relief to find out how to help their child, thus re-evaluating their own parenting skills. This gives children the opportunity to face their problems with the family that is primarily the source of their well-being or suffering. In this way, a context will be created in which children, while experiencing their own skills as autonomous individuals capable of social coexistence, may discover the possibility of explaining their problems and may see the opening up of new ways of understanding. The widened context also allows parents to understand, in participating in their child's play, the psychological aspects underlying eating and evacuative conduct, favouring, with appropriate interventions, the emergence of family harmony. This may happen more easily when parents have adequate personal skills, while a more complex therapeutic project may be required when these skills are seriously compromised (such as, for example, a prolonged PC intervention over time, an intervention only with the child and a space to provide support to parents).

4. Focal Play-Therapy and narrative play

As already highlighted, FPT carried out in PC can be placed in the current clinical context, where increasing attention is paid to the narrative dimension of the young patients in their family context.

At this point, it would good to point out some fundamental aspects about play and narrative play underlined by Dina Vallino (2004; 2009; 2012):

- Play is located at the crossroads of the adult's recognition of the child, it is the way the infant tries to exist with the other's help.
- In child psychoanalysis, through symbolic play, conscious and unconscious fantasy and the Imaginary Place, contextual to the representation of the fantasies, are confirmed as fundamental cognitive and affective functions (Vallino 1998).
- Symbolic play, supported by the *personification* process (Klein 1929),[3] manages to develop into narrative play when the child's imagination is nourished by the *reverie* activity and the sense of responsibility of the adult, who helps to give a sense of continuity to the narrative.
- With narrative play, Dina Vallino intends a wide range of activities through which children spontaneously draw on their imagination to externalize, with allegories, metaphors and symbols, a new version of their internal experiences and external events, which they place in a concrete space, for a specific time, through sketches and small narrations.
- Narrative play does not require verbalized interpretations, but only a *narrative interpretation*, which often has the sole purpose of rekindling the momentum of play, of showing some new aspects of it.

Examples of this are some of the therapist's sentences presented in the clinical case of Aldo in this chapter. Specifically, the therapist, through their own character named Lewie, comments on the speed of Aldo's car: "You're so fast, little car! Who knows where you get all that energy from?" Aldo replies: "it's because I fill up with petrol!", inserting a pump (he himself built with playdough) into the tank of the car. The parents try to help him, suggesting, however, to do this for him in his stead. The therapist/Lewie intervenes saying (narrative interpretation): "so many suggestions! ... how confusing! ... we could do that mom and dad help soften the playdough, ... and then Aldo makes the petrol pump, as he is very able to build it by himself!"

After these clarifications, some fundamental aspects of FPT in PC, already partially highlighted (Trombini 2010; 2011), will be further expanded upon.

A first aspect regards the role of the therapist, who becomes a living and concrete presence within the narrative. In fact, at first the therapist presents, giving it voice, the playdough puppet Lewie which carries out the eating–evacuation sequence. The therapist then retreats to the background, to allow the child to project his psychic contents. However, the therapist does not give the child the puppet, which therefore remains on the table and to which the therapist continues to give voice: commenting, for example, on what happens in the child's narrative play and/or suggesting to model other characters, companions in the story that is being built starting from this new reference framework.

In this way Lewie is characterized as the one who, through its behaviour, highlights the characteristics of autonomy in the relationship with food and evacuative functions. But it also enables the representation of the therapist as a "somewhat special companion" able to accompany the child in that Imaginary Place, where everything is possible and where the most horrible ideas can be embodied in frightening monsters, which may, however, be defeated: a screen on which to project aspects of the soul otherwise not perceivable. In this way the characters of the Imaginary Place, invented in the encounter between the child and the analyst in the presence of the parents, lend themselves to giving voice to terrors that the child is unable to approach or to changes that the child is unable to plan (Vallino, 1998, 2000, 2009).

Therefore, therapists, through Lewie, can express their function as observers, comforters, companions, *Narrators within the Narration.*

As an example, a summary is offered of some passages of the consultation – already extensively presented elsewhere (Trombini 2011) – with Cloe (two years and three months) and her parents, who contact the therapist for their daughter's eating problems. This example highlights the function of the therapist–narrator from as early as the first meeting.

As soon as Cloe arrives she enthusiastically agrees to play with the play dough, personally suggesting the name "Phil" for the playdough puppet the therapist is modelling. The father intervenes by inviting his daughter to say its name, the place where it lives and what it must say if it gets lost. Cloe responds with accelerated language, a little stereotyped and charming, continuing to be interested in Phil, who she puts to bed. The father suggests giving Phil a belly massage, as he himself gives the girl before putting her to bed. At this point Cloe, determined, leaves the game and lies down under the table. Her mum urges her to come out, but the girl doesn't move and says: "I'm in bed!"

The therapist waits a little and then, taking the playdough doll, asks: "Can I come sleep with you?" Cloe opens up in a smile: "Mum, do you see the little boy is coming to sleep with me!" She then comes out from under the table accompanied by the puppet Phil/therapist to return to play on the table. The therapist then proposes the FPT sequence, preparing together with the child, who actively participates, the meatballs with which to feed Phil which, when its stomach is full, goes to evacuate. The mother offers to make plates and forks which Cloe is happy to accept. The father stands up, looks around, is unable to participate, while the mother is particularly involved in the narration. At the end of the session Cloe observes her hands, green with playdough. The therapist exclaims: "mine are green too, because we played!". The mother also shows hers, green, smiling. Cloe then turns to her dad, who has clean hands, and with hers she dirties the father's, who smiles. The girl then wants us all to go to the bathroom to wash our hands.

A second aspect concerns the role of the parent. In fact, from a methodological point of view, the use of playdough allows the therapist (through Lewie) not only to be narrator within the narration, but also to favour the parent's function as observer, comforter, companion within the narration, setting up other playdough characters for the parent. In this way, the parents are encouraged, through their characters, to become players too, as will be shown in the clinical vignettes that will be presented later.

A third aspect concerns the possibility for the therapist to observe the ways in which parents and their child play, as they favour or hinder the therapeutic process (Trombini & Trombini 2007). Specifically, parenting behaviour "favouring" play is characterized by tolerant patience, collaboration, offers of support, suggestions aligned with the creative intentions of the child, an enthusiasm confident in the child's productivity. While behaviours "hindering" play are characterized by impositions rather than suggestions, distracting or off-topic interventions, disinterest and/or self-exclusion from the scene of play.

The clinical example of Cloe, cited above, highlights the mother's behaviour favouring the game and the father's hindering behaviour during the first session. It also highlights Cloe's extraordinary ability to want and be able to involve her father in the group activity, first by dirtying his hands and then inviting everyone to wash their hands.

5. "Getting in the game" with children and parents through Focal Play-Therapy: clinical vignettes[4]

Focal Play-Therapy constitutes the method by which parents and children with eating and evacuation disorders are welcomed in the Psychological Consultation Service for children and parents, at the Department of Psychology of the University of Bologna. This service makes use of the collaboration of psychotherapists with psychoanalytic training, all experts in the above-mentioned methodology.

The prolonged sharing of the suffering of children and parents and the constant supervision work, shared by the author, deeply and over a long time, with Dina Vallino and the colleagues of the supervision group on PC, motivates the need for further reflections here, accompanied by clinical material, which will be presented in the form of bullet-points.

- By showing the FPT sequence, the therapist (T) "tells" the child and the parents, introducing the narrative plan, about the child's problem.
- At the end of the first session, in which PC is presented, focused on observing the child's play and behaviour, the parents frequently ask how to explain to their child the reason for going to the therapist. The author lets the parents themselves choose how to talk to the child and what to talk about. When the child with the parents is then welcomed, the FPT sequence is used as an organized starting point to explain the problem for which the child and parents have come to the therapist. The parents feel relieved and understood.
- In this regard, the author recalls the words of a father: "through the proposed game, you hit the problem on its head, and caught the attention of my son." In other words, it is evident how the FPT sequence enables one to face the child's problem, through being able to speak with both the child and the parents in a lighter emotional climate.
- During the PC meetings, the FPT sequence is repeated several times, in the sense that it is repeated both within the same session and/or in subsequent sessions and is alternated with the narrative ideas that gradually emerge during the session. The therapist's suggestion to repeat the sequence keeps the attention focused on the problem of the child; it allows the children to explain, in their own personal ways, their psychic contents. It also allows the therapist to discriminate when the children repetitively perform the sequence compared to when, supported by the therapist and the collaborative attitude of the parents, they instead manage to find creative ways towards a gradual resolution of their problems.

5.1 Clinical vignette

Aldo (age 3 years, 10 months), whose little brother was recently born, has tantrums during meals with his parents and, according to them for no apparent reason, often stops eating and leaves the table. In addition, since his diaper was removed (when he was 2 years and 6 months), he soils his pants: during the day he pees in the toilet, but he stubbornly refuses to evacuate his faeces in the toilet or to wear a nappy.

Aldo is a lively, nice, attentive child. In the first session he introduces himself, showing how he can jump and run fast.

Aldo brought along with him two toy cars which he uses to make acrobatic evolutions. In the therapist's room Aldo looks with interest at the playdough box. The therapist suggests they play with it and builds Lewie (L).

Aldo looks amused: the therapist continues by presenting the sequence. Aldo is very careful and asks that the therapist/Lewie goes through the sequence several times, but without taking part in it directly. He then returns to excitedly show how his toy car "runs fast, up into the sky". The parents look at him pleased: the father tends to get him excited by continuously suggesting new game activities, to then block his liveliness (don't speak so loudly, ... sit, ... wait ...).

The therapist (T)/L comments "You're so fast, little car! Who knows where you get all that energy from?" Aldo replies: "it's because I fill up with petrol!", inserting a pump (he himself built with playdough) into the tank of the car. The parents try to help him, but suggesting they do things in his stead. The father also continues to make distracting game suggestions ("why don't we make another truck as well?"). T/L intervenes saying: "so many suggestions! ... how confusing! ... we could do that mom and dad help soften the playdough, ... and then Aldo makes the petrol pump, as he is very able to build it by himself!"

In the second session, Aldo's cars run on a circuit set up on the table. L looks at them with amusement and at the end of the races he comments: "It's so nice to watch these races ... now that they are over I am hungry ... shall we have a snack?" Aldo nods. T/L eats and then evacuates; Aldo "feeds" his cars with "petrol" with his petrol pump, which then "emits smoke" (built with playdough and positioned by Aldo in the back of his cars).

In the following session Aldo places alongside his toy cars a small robot, which he wants to build with playdough, and which becomes the main character of the story, accompanied by L and other playdough characters held by his parents, now much more in line with Aldo's play proposals. During this session Aldo personally feeds his robot and makes it evacuate in the toilet together with L.

5.1.1 Comment

The parents were helped both by the therapist/Lewie's suggestions during the play sessions and by the reflections shared during the sessions without Aldo, during which it was possible to talk about the inappropriateness of certain contradictory parental requests (which excite and block) and about Aldo's need to be able to act autonomously, especially with regard to eating and evacuation without constant pressing requests from his parents, also worried in this period by the management of two young children, the second of which had just been born.

In the following two sessions Aldo and his parents took part with pleasure in the narrative plot in which, with a family of robots as protagonists, each of them, through their own character, performed, in harmony with the other members, pleasant daily tasks (having lunch, going to the park to play, going to sleep). At the same time, the problems manifested by Aldo in terms of his eating and evacuating behaviour were completely resolved.

5.1.2 When and how to involve parents

It has already been underlined how in FPT in PC the parents, taking part in their children's play, can grasp the latter's real interests expressed in it, and can, in greater contact with their children, find out how to help them, thus re-evaluating their own parenting skills. The child is, however, the primary focus of the therapist's (T) attention.

Therefore the T first encourages the participatory behaviour of the parents, after asking the child, with phrases like: "shall we get help from mom and dad to soften the playdough to prepare the meatballs (or other foods)?". Only later does the T ask the child: "can we also give mom and dad a character so that they can play with us?", allowing the child to suggest the characters for the parents, who go from being participating spectators to becoming players themselves. This allows the therapists to better observe the parenting behaviour, favouring or hindering the child's narration, to then modulate their interventions inside and outside the narrative plane.

5.2 Clinical vignette

Roberto's case – already briefly presented in Trombini (2010) – shows the role of the therapist and the parents within the narrative plane. Specifically, in this clinical vignette parental behaviours which are characterized by aspects that hinder play are highlighted. These characteristics, deeply rooted in the parents' culture of origin, will bear heavily on the therapeutic process, which will be interrupted by them before achieving complete self-regulation of the child's eating behaviour.

Roberto (Rb) is four years of age: he was born prematurely (a birthweight of 1140 grams), in the middle of the sixth month of pregnancy. Food has never given him pleasure and his mother needs to spoon-feed him to make him eat, even for an hour and a half, in front of the TV to try to distract him. These behaviours are also present in school, a place where Rb is shy and lonely. On returning home he abandons himself to sucking on his pillow, lying on his bed: his mother, irritated, comments that "thanks to this, he gets rid of hunger and thirst".

Rb is described by his parents as a child who plays repetitive games, putting objects in a row and tying them together. The parents are exasperated by their son's behaviour and the mother points out that, when she gives him milk in the bottle in the morning, he does not grab hold of it and drops his arms on the table, thus expressing his passive protest. When his mother was hospitalized to give birth to his little sister (now one year of age), Rb feared that he would never see her again and subsequently became seriously and repeatedly ill with bronchitis that forced him to stay home from nursery.

I suggest a participated consultation with Rb and his parents which will continue for 15 sessions.

Rb presents himself from the beginning as an alert and curious child, not at all shy, capable of proposing and continuing, even if with a polite tone, a narration of his in a decisive and active way, which always involves both mom and dad.

In the first session, Rb starts a game in which, in a serious and busy way, he loads many playdough balls built by him on a truck, commenting: "they look like small meatballs". The Therapist (T), through Lewie, observes Rb's efforts with curiosity and attention and finds a way to propose the FPT sequence by making L say: "So much work with all these balls/meatballs ... now I would really like to have a snack!" Rb accepts and excitedly feeds L personally. Immediately the mother enters the game and goes against him asking to have food for herself; the T intervenes: "we are playing it is L who wants to have a snack!"

In the following sessions Rb plays out some recurring narrative ideas. He prepares foods with which he fills trains and trucks. He says of himself: "I am a waiter carrying sweets for mom and dad." Rb plays being a cook who prepares omelettes and who loves to eat sweets, but only towards the end of the session, after a long preparation. Rb is a child/cook who models and controls, but the parents, even if they try to play his game, interfere and oppress him.

In fact, during the sessions the mother makes suggestions that are not aligned with the child's creative narrative, making comments that remain on the concrete level of everyday life. During the FPT sequence, Rb also proposes other recurring themes: rescue trains appear, fire trucks that put out the fires produced by the stove fire. The father intervenes mainly with intrusive behaviours: he proposes themes of his own, such as sticking a playdough moustache on his son's train. The T, during a meeting with the parents only, comments: "it is as if each of you wants to follow your own project." The father replies: "everyone wants to play his game. With Rb, I do this almost on purpose." The T stresses that it is important to reflect on the need, in playing together, to try to also understand the purpose of the other and to allow time for the other to manifest it.

It emerges that the origin of this behaviour in the parents can be traced back to what their idea is in respect to their educational role, with strong implications tied to their culture of origin: being parent–guide is seen as a priority. However, they also understand the need to activate a process of transformation of their attitude towards the needs of Rb. Therefore during the meetings the T directs the parents' attention towards respecting Rb's times and ways to express himself, highlighting his creative abilities to self-regulate. At the same time, the T makes Rb's desire to remain in emotional contact with both parents, spontaneously following their guidance–proposals, emerge. Consequently, during the sessions, the mother describes herself as calmer and more capable of tolerating the times and rhythms of Rb, while the father spends more time with his son and comments "we should let him do things without discouraging him".

There were improvements on the level of family relationships and eating behaviour: during meals Rb was now made to sit at the table with his sister (and no longer alone) and he ate with greater autonomy (no longer spoon-fed).

However, at the fourteenth session, only with the parents, the father surprised the T by suddenly communicating his intention to suspend the therapy. This appeared to be connected to his deep-rooted thought that "being parents means that it is up to us to be guides in teaching". They declared themselves very satisfied with the progress made and confident that they could continue to help their child on their own. An attitude of implicit rivalry of the father towards the function of the T as promoter and support of the son's autonomy seemed to emerge. However, the father's strong need to be recognized in his will and ability to manage by himself in his parenting role became evident. The T therefore decided to underline how this motivation for autonomy characterized, but above all was common to, both parents and the child. The T also stressed that this motivation, which emerged during the sessions, allowed them, the parents, to activate behaviours that were more respectful of the need for autonomy of Rb and therefore to be able to reach an increased family harmony.

In the following, last, meeting with parents and Rb, the child had the opportunity to express what he felt and thought through play: preparing a "shower that washes all", he communicated his perception of how the T had washed his parents' anxiety and at the same time supported his abilities, through the construction of a "new railway, with a train that repairs itself, but which still needs time".

In saying good-bye to Rb and his parents, the T summarized what had emerged and explained: "in this room we all played together games that were a bit special ... in which mom and dad learned to play better with him. Now you can continue at home, following the proposals of Rb, who is very capable of narrating while playing, but above all he is eager to do it together with his parents."

6. Conclusive thoughts

Focal Play-Therapy is a methodology that enables, in the here and now of the meeting with child and parents, the listening and the identification of the experiences and the problems underlying the symptoms related to food and eating, while also enabling the reactivation, with the support of the therapist, of the creative means through which parents and children manage to proceed together along developmental paths.

It is therefore a methodology that is part of the underlying construct of the *Mindful Emotion Regulation Approach*, since it allows the clinician to pay special attention to the here and now, in order to promote in the family, as the editors of the volume point out, the presence of an accepting, non-judgemental attitude capable of adequately regulating emerging emotions. In this regard, Focal Play-Therapy with the child and the parents allows the former to see the latter's constructive attitudes, emerging during therapy, as they develop. Similarly, parents can observe the transformations of the child as they occur and can therefore realize that the transformation that takes place is also the result of their active collaboration, in which their understanding of the needs of their child plays a fundamental role.

Specifically, Focal Play-Therapy, by proposing a setting with rules, constitutes an organized starting point, capable of promoting the achievement of self-managed and self-regulated child behaviours, integrated into a harmonious family life. It also allows parents to feel valued in their parenting skills. In this way, parents can grasp the children's real interests expressed in the game, their non-verbal way of expressing them, their desires, fears and angers. In the vision of the parents, the child who refuses to eat is no longer just a body-organism that needs to feed itself, which is risking its own health. Eating behaviour is no longer only perceived on a concrete level: it is now possible to interpret it in its psychological meaning. The setting promotes respect for the child's way of playing and the possibility of playing with the child without intrusive and directive attitudes. In this context, parents, who are incentivized to become players as well, have the opportunity to experience their ability to play and try out a pleasant participation. Going along with the game, they can focus on what is going on, also using their own imagination. They can thus recover their playful and creative child self, alongside the observational aspects of their adult self. This may happen more easily when parents already have these personal skills, while a more complex therapeutic project is required when these skills are seriously compromised.

To conclude, some aspects should be highlighted.

What does the use of playdough, privileged material of FPT, add to that of other toys present in a therapist's room (family characters, animals ...) in setting off the narrative plane?

Playdough is a pliable substance particularly appreciated in preschool age, which harks back to the pleasure of manipulating, creating, destroying, transforming and which allows one to express deep feelings. Playdough therefore lends itself very well to giving voice to changing, ambivalent, aggressive, restorative feelings, such as those that support eating and evacuative symptoms.

For example, the young patient may express feelings of anger by violently crushing Lewie. The Therapist, who does not lose his role as narrator within the narration, can give voice to what is happening, making Lewie speak: "ouch, ouch I'm all bruised, maybe the one who hit me was really angry!" This allows the child to feel understood and simultaneously offers the opportunity to continue the narration, together with the therapist. Many times, in fact, in these cases, the narration resumes with the exhortation of the young patient: "now you make Lewie's head and arms again because we have to keep playing!"

Playdough also encourages the involvement of the parent as a player.

With regard to this involvement, there are fathers who express their diffi-culty in taking part in the game proposed by their daughter with dolls and toy pots and pans, while they are happily involved in preparing playdough meatballs for the snack of the daughter's doll during the FPT. Similar situa-tions can occur with mothers of boys who mainly love to play with toy cars. An example of this is Aldo's mother who was able to join the game by setting up, using the playdough, other petrol pumps to refuel the cars and by orga-nizing the garage to let the cars rest at night.

As for the modalities of play that might favour or hinder the child's narra-tion, the use of playdough facilitates the observation of the therapist also regarding the great pleasure or the excessive annoyance of the parent in the manipulation. Obstructive modalities are present for example when parents become absorbed by their own playdough creation: they do not prepare a simple meatball, but a spectacular multi-layered and multi-coloured sandwich (completely realistic), which makes them lose sight of the times and contents of the narration taking place, proposed by the child. Or when the parents ask the children to wash their hands after having manipulated the playdough, so as not to dirty their own clothes, or ask the therapist if they themselves can wash their hands before leaving the consultation room.

Finally, through playdough one can create anything: characters and objects that are not present among the ones that are usually in the child psychother-apy room, fantastical characters and completely specific ones, arising from the therapeutic context. In this regard, the children ask to take home some playdough characters or small shapeless pieces "to play with mom and dad": the desire for continuity between the therapeutic context and the daily family emotional atmosphere is evident. In some cases the children bring the play-dough characters back in the following session, to continue the narration. In others, it is the parents who inform the therapist that they have purchased more playdough to play at home with their child.

With playdough, psychic changes and transformations can be made evident and tangible: both through the characters represented (as in the case of a small patient who stretched the body of his playdough baby, to show that he "had grown up"); both through the ways in which the playdough is manipu-lated by the child (in a formless or more articulated way).

These features also make playdough particularly useful to keep the field delimited and focus the narrative attention of children and parents who, too often, in the current context, are immersed in a daily life in which objects (toys) risk invading their space, hindering or breaking up narrative plots.

Highlights

• The chapter presented "Focal Play-Therapy" (FPT) as a specific pre-ventive–therapeutic intervention that enables one to deal with eating

disorders in preschool age with parents and children, through a methodology that facilitates attention to what happens in the here and now,
offering an opportunity to show parents "how to be together" with their
children in the game, observing and listening to them.

- FPT is implemented in the context of the Participated Consultation
  intervention developed by Dina Vallino. Therefore the structure of the
  meetings consists of the alternation of play sessions with the child and
  parents and meetings only with the parental couple, in which the therapist returns to the narrative elements that emerged during the sessions of
  shared play and the emotions underlying it.
- By placing the children at its centre, FPT highlights their characteristics
  of autonomy in the relationship with food and evacuative contents and
  allows parents to take part in their children's play and to grasp their real
  interests expressed in it, their desires, fears and angers.
- In the FPT sessions, the therapist proposes a temporal sequence where
  the protagonist is a playdough puppet (Lewie). The playdough used in
  the game is particularly suitable because it is a pliable material that harks
  back to the pleasure of manipulating, creating, destroying, transforming,
  which allows the child to express deep experiences and which also favours
  the involvement of the parent as a player.
- After establishing a warm and friendly contact with the child, the therapist guides Lewie in carrying out the physiological functions of feeding
  and evacuation. In this way, the therapist clarifies the meaning of these
  physiological functions by integrating nutrition and evacuation as part of
  a single process, so as to configure them in their natural aspect.
- The therapist then gradually withdraws into the background, allowing the
  children to externalize and project their psychic contents, in particular
  those of an aggressive type, into their play. The therapist intervenes, when
  appropriate, with comments expressed in a simple way and only referring
  to what takes place in the events of the game, or with suggestions on
  possible alternative solutions to the events being staged.
- FPT with child and parents therefore allows one to identify the problems
  underlying the feeding symptoms and to promote in parents an attitude
  capable of adequately regulating emerging emotions.
- By proposing a setting with rules, FPT constitutes an organized starting
  point, capable of promoting the achievement of self-managed and self-
  regulated child behaviours, integrated into a harmonious family life.

Notes

1 In the request to do things by themselves, the children's experiences are structured
   around three polarities: (1) the subject, source of the action; (2) the physical object,
   on which the action is directed; (3) the adult, with whom to negotiate roles. With
   these behaviours the child shows an ability to control complex dynamics. In fact,

faced with an intervention by the adult who tries to help out with the target action, the child does not lose sight of the purpose that animates him or the human partner with whom he continues to communicate (Arfelli Galli 2006).

2 Vallino writes (2009, p. 44): "Participated Consultation sessions are, from my point of view, an early psychoanalysis in the sense that parents are encouraged to take care of their young children taking into account their emotional mind and their personality. A type of attention towards the child that implies the parents' elaboration of their misunderstanding (... which prevents them from understanding the child's signals, causing inadequate responses) and of the pathological projective identification towards the child. By becoming 'participating observers' of the relationship between themselves and their child, parents will become able to grasp their child's sensitivity and mental capacity, which will allow them to be, with the analyst, the protagonists of a psychoanalytical study.

In Participated Consultation, no evaluation by the analyst is useful, with regard to the parents' skills, as long as the analyst does not have the means to observe them in action, the parents with their child."

3 Klein (1929) explained, in "Personification in the play of children", that "one (of the) principal mechanism in games (is the one) in which different characters are invented and allotted by the child. My object in the present paper is to discuss this mechanism in more detail and also to illustrate ... the relation between the 'characters' or personifications introduced by them into these games and the element of wish-fulfilment".

"In the case of my little patient, Erna, who was six years old when we began the treatment, a severe obsessional neurosis marked a paranoia which was revealed after a considerable amount of analysis. In her play Erna often made me be a child, while she was the mother or a teacher. I then had to undergo fantastic tortures and humiliations. If in the game anyone treated me kindly, it generally turned out that the kindness was only simulated ... I myself, in the role of the child, had constantly to spy upon and torment the others. Often Erna herself played the part of the child. Then the game generally ended in her escaping the persecutions (on these occasions the 'child' was good), becoming rich and powerful, being made a queen and taking a cruel revenge on her persecutors."

4 All clinical cases presented in the chapter were personally followed by Elena Trombini at the Psychological Consultation Service for children and parents (Department of Psychology, University of Bologna), which she personally set up and currently directs.

Chapter 6

Food selectivity and pre-adolescence

Anna Maria Delogu

1. Pre-adolescence: a matter of boundaries

The definition of pre-adolescence, as a specific developmental phase, appears somewhat critical and unclear (Bosi & Zavattini 1982), leaving room for it to be determined *by difference*: no longer childhood and not yet adolescence. The adoption of a chronological criterion or a biological one that takes into account the somatic transformations that occur in this period may be rather simplistic, missing its specificity on the psychological level (Blos 1979).

Eccles (1999), analysing development between the ages of 6 and 14, proposes a distinction in two phases, middle childhood (approximately 6–10 years of age) and early adolescence (approximately 11–14 years of age), each of which appears to be characterized by deep biological, cognitive and relational changes. The former corresponds to what Erikson (1959) defined as the period of *industry vs. inferiority* where the range of relationships expands outside the family context and during which positive experiences enable the child to build a sense of competence; failed experiences will instead bring a sense of inadequacy and inferiority. Three factors contribute to the adequate completion of this developmental phase, namely the cognitive changes that bring about a greater ability to reflect on oneself and to grasp others' perspectives, the expansion of social relationships with greater investment on relationships outside the family and the exposure to social confrontation in the school context and in the group of peers. In early adolescence, the physiological changes connected to puberty occur and the process of building one's own identity as an autonomous individual begins, the phase of *identity vs. role confusion*, according to Erikson (1959), during which specific tasks are related to restructuring one's own body image following the pubertal somatic changes and the process of separation–individuation with respect to the parental figures.

Kerns (2008) speaks of middle childhood, referring to children between 7 and 12 years of age, highlighting the children's tendency to continue searching for available attachment figures, while recognizing the decreasingly exclusive value of this relationship. Attachment security, in fact, continues to act as a functional factor for exploration which, in this specific period of development, can be understood in a broad sense as the possibility of "exploring" new relationships and the emotions associated with physical, cognitive and social changes.[1] It is in this specific developmental period that the perception of one's own body and the satisfaction/dissatisfaction with one's own body image become particularly relevant and can act as risk factors with respect to the onset of an eating disorder (Menzel et al. 2010; Thompson & Stice 2001).

2. Food selectivity: brief nosographic notes

The intake of a limited range of foods during childhood is often a source of concern for parents as it is linked to the ideas of an incorrect intake of nutrients and of possible repercussions on physical development, as well as to the questioning of the relationship itself.

Children can show an apparent aversion to or avoidance of certain foods based on their consistency, colour, appearance or smell, up to selecting them based on the type of packaging or brand or temperature. Bryant-Waugh, Markham, Kreipe and Walsh (2010) underline the terms used to describe the eating behaviour of these children, distinguishing between *selective eating*, understood as the tendency to eat a very limited range of foods, *perseverant eaters*, those individuals who tend to eat through means specific to a previous developmental phase, *food neophobia*, that is the aversion to trying new foods to broaden one's own eating repertoire and *sensory food refusal*. Food selectivity is often already present in early childhood and is distinguished from neophobias because it concerns the refusal of foods that are familiar to the child. These problems, often referred to as *picky or fussy eating*, are more frequent in preschool age, with a peak incidence at the age of six, and can last up to the age of 11 with similar characteristics in childhood and pre-adolescence (Cardona Cano et al. 2015; Jacobi, Schmitz, & Stewart 2008; Lam 2015; Mascola, Bryson, & Agras 2010; Taylor, Wernimont, Northstone, & Emmett 2015).[2] Furthermore, this kind of behaviour is associated with a greater risk of not gaining weight and eating practices that are adequate with respect to chronological age, a greater probability of manifesting an eating disorder (ED) (Cate, Khademi, Judd, & Miller 2013) and a high level of conflict in the mother–child relationship (Tharner et al. 2014). Interestingly, a recent attempt to define *picky eating* in operational terms has led to the identification of a specific profile in which individual and family factors are intertwined. Tharner et al. (2014) in fact found an eating behaviour profile characterized by fussiness, slowness in eating and reactivity to satiety in combination with poor pleasure derived from eating and a greater sensitivity to food. A significant correlation between low family income and selective eating behaviour was also highlighted. A short breastfeeding period,[3] low variety of foods in the mother's diet and pressure to eat by the parents were indicated as factors that could influence food selectivity during childhood (Galloway, Lee, & Birch 2003; Galloway, Fiorito, Lee, & Birch 2005).

Some studies have focused on the link between food selectivity and specific individual characteristics of the child, such as anxiety and increased sensitivity to sensory stimuli (Bryant-Waugh, Markham, Kreipe, & Walsh 2010); in particular, the child's anxiety seems to significantly predict the manifestation of eating difficulties, including food aversion and neophobias, up to the later onset of eating disorders in adolescence. In addition to this, a comorbidity between food selectivity, anxiety and obsessive–compulsive behaviours (in situations related or unrelated to nutrition) is sometimes found (Farrow & Coulthard 2012), thus describing the possible emergence of a more complex and extensive pattern of individual risk. An example of this is given by the fact that the processes of regulation, intended as skills learned within the early relationship between mother and child, also include an inevitable reference to a neurobiological component, which contributes to defining the child's specificity, mediating – among others – the link between anxiety and selective behaviour.

In this direction, the emotional structure of the mother, and of caregivers in general, appears to be of fundamental importance since it represents the malleable component, the influence of which can determine different outcomes depending on the quality of the relationship with the child and, therefore, towards an adequate – or inadequate – attunement to the child's physical and emotional needs. If the mother experiences anxiety or depression she will be less responsive in the feeding interaction, adopting a more controlling style that could act as a risk factor with respect to the child developing a selective eating behaviour (Hafstad, Abebe, Torgersen, & von Soest 2013). This controlling style seems to determine an inhibition of the child's exploratory capacity, expressed through selectivity, which reinforces and amplifies the emotional experience of the caregiver.

Although research mainly focused either on infancy, in an attempt to trace early risk factors, or on adolescence/adulthood – to understand and treat more structured psychopathological patterns – from a clinical point of view it is not uncommon to observe that even the intermediate phases represent important developmental turning points for children and, in some cases, moments when to intervene before behaviours become organized in a more stable and lasting manner. In fact, clinical experience underlines the persistence, if not the intensification of conflict with the increase in age of children as well as the relevance of aspects connected to the parent–child relationship in the transition from childhood to the next phase, pre-adolescence, which brings about different developmental tasks for both children and parents.

3. Family-based interventions

Empirical research has shown the effectiveness of family interventions in the treatment of eating disorders, confirming and reinforcing what had emerged from the pioneering work of Salvador Minuchin and Mara Selvini Palazzoli

(Eisler, le Grange, & Asen 2006). These contributions emphasized the transactional modalities and relational dynamics that occur in families of anorexic patients (Minuchin et al. 1980; Selvini Palazzoli, Cirillo, Selvini, & Sorrentino 1988, 1998) but are not specific to families where a member manifests an eating disorder nor can they be considered causal factors (le Grange et al. 2009). Turning this perspective around, it is true that the presence of a member with an eating disorder affects family life (Nielsen & Barà-Carrill 2006) and that working therapeutically with all family members can lead to a change in the functioning of the whole family nucleus (Eisler et al. 2000).

Working with families means interacting with an interpersonal system governed by rules of interaction (Jackson 1977), the constituent elements of which are both the members that make it up and the reciprocal relationships they build. Minuchin (1976) defines the family as "the invisible set of functional demands that determines the ways in which family members interact", boundaries and principles of regulation among which the maintenance of homeostasis (internal balance) of the family, through the development of relationship "rules",[4] takes on particular importance.

The structural model focuses on family organization: the family system contains subsystems, that is "aggregations of particular members linked by a close relationship; by definition they have implicit 'boundaries' that exclude others" (Minuchin, Reiter, & Borda 2013, p. 67). Examples of this are the parental couple, which is also a marital couple, the filial subsystem as well as the subsystems that are defined by the members' belonging to the same gender. The boundaries, however, need to maintain a degree of flexibility, to guarantee on the one hand transition of information and affects and on the other hand autonomy, specificity of roles and processes of differentiation[5] (Onnis 2004). The affiliations defined by the subsystems can become "coalitions, when certain family members unite to contest or attack other members. When intergenerational coalitions appear, they are often an expression of pathology and a source of tension" (Minuchin, Reiter, & Borda 2013, p. 67). Through the exploration of the family system and of its subsystems it is possible to understand the role of each member with respect to the dysfunctional, symptomatic model brought into therapy, thus shifting the focus from the designated patient to the system as a whole.

If it is true that these concepts guide clinical practice in a well-established way, scientific contributions related to the effectiveness of family therapy in the treatment of eating disorders are influenced by two factors: first, empirical studies mainly focus on a specific population of patients, i.e., female adolescents with anorexia nervosa (Abbate Daga et al. 2011; Carr 2014; Eisler, le Grange, & Asen 2006);[6] secondly, the intervention models are heterogeneous, refer to different theoretical frameworks and tend towards the integration of multiple perspectives.

Several studies, however, have highlighted the efficacy of family-based therapy (FBT)[7] in the treatment of anorexia nervosa (Dare, Eisler, Russell, &

Szmukler 1990; Lock & le Grange 2001; 2013). This intervention perspective can be defined as the outcome of the integration of the previous models of family treatments (Lock & le Grange 2013) and focuses on the resources and abilities that parents possess and can activate to help their child (Murray, Griffiths, & le Grange 2014).

While recognizing the validity of *evidence-based* interventions such as FBT in the treatment of eating disorders, it is crucial to think of an *integrated* model that enables the understanding of the family context in structural and representational terms, promoting and using mentalization and *mindfulness* processes as possible activators of change. The term "mentalization" indicates a process, and not a mental state or static individual characteristics, which usually occurs without specific awareness; mentalizing means explicitly thinking about mental states and understanding their relationship with feelings and behaviours. Mentalization and the fullness of mental awareness can be defined as

> processes of "disembedding" [...] Throughout our lives, mentalizing has the potential to free us from embeddedness in the internal world and external reality by fostering awareness of the interpretive depth and representational nature of subjective experience in ourselves and others.
>
> (Wallin 2007, p. 463)

This process is fundamental with respect to understanding and interpreting the behaviour of the other as well as one's own and it becomes extremely relevant when working with families. The family system is in fact configured as a complex structure in which it is possible to recognize networks of relationships and representations that are related to a constant dialogue between the *interpersonal* and *intrapsychic* dimensions. It could be said that mentalization in the context of a family-based intervention enables the disembedding from the external (behaviours, interactions, symptomatic aspects) and internal reality of each member to render explicit and connect each one's subjective experience so as to enable a new understanding of the family's organization.

The *mentalization-based treatment for families* (MBT-F; Asen & Fonagy 2012), in line with what was highlighted above, promotes awareness of the impact of one's own thoughts, feelings and actions on the other, the ability to take on a confident, humble and playful attitude, the belief that change is possible, the acceptance of responsibility, as well as forgiveness, intended as the ability to reinterpret other individuals' actions on the basis of an understanding and acceptance of their mental states. The clinician can activate reflection on these aspects through *curiosity*, understood as a means that can "challenge" the family's certainties that hinder change, explore alternatives and use the content to understand the process, highlighting the *circularity*, that is the concatenation of a series of family system states, through the exploration of the subjective experiences of each member of the family (Malagoli Togliatti, & Cotugno 1996; Minuchin, Reiter, & Borda 2013).

Interventions focused on mentalization are used both in family and individual therapy and also have similarities with other intervention models, including Dialectical Behaviour Therapy (DBT; Linehan 1987).[8] Perepletchikova and Goodman (2014) compared DBT and MBT in the treatment of pre-adolescents with emotional and behavioural problems, highlighting similarities and differences. Both interventions emphasize the *present moment* as current experience and promote closeness, but also differentiation of mental states; DBT and MBT, however, differ in the interpretation of the factors at the origin of the identified problems: the first perspective considers symptomatological aspects as arising from skill deficits, inhibition of emotions, challenging environmental circumstances and problematic beliefs and expectations; the second perspective sees the problematic aspects as arising from difficulties in the mentalization process. As one would expect, these divergences lead to different therapeutic techniques, despite being united by the objective of promoting the acquisition of self-regulation skills and an improvement in functioning.

Attention focused on the present moment clearly brings to mind the definition of *mindfulness*, intended as the ability to focus, intentionally, on one's own sensorial, cognitive and emotional experience, without judging any one part of it (Kabat-Zinn 1994). Germer (2005) succinctly defines it as awareness and acceptance of the present moment. Several contributions emphasize the role of *mindfulness* in relation to emotion regulation processes connected to various psychopathological manifestations (Mikulincer & Shaver, 2008). Recently, Pepping, O'Donovan, Zimmer-Gembeck and Hanisch (2014), for example, highlighted the mediating role of mindfulness in the relationship between insecure attachment and eating behaviour pathology, in a sample of women aged between 17 and 41 and, in particular, between the anxiety and avoidance related to attachment and the eating disorder. From the concept of *mindfulness* derives that of *mindful eating*, that is "a non-judgmental awareness of the physical and emotional sensations associated with eating" (Framson et al. 2009), which was operationalized in the context of interventions aimed at treating *binge eating disorder* (Mindfulness-Based Eating Awareness Training – MB-EAT; Kristeller, Baer, & Wolever 2006; Kristeller & Hallett 1999; Kristeller & Wolever 2011; Wolever & Best 2009) in which food takes on the function of emotion regulator and in which one can observe a dysregulation of the mechanisms tied to hunger and satiety. These aspects are present, albeit in a different way, even in patients with restrictive eating behaviours (Albers 2011).

The concept of *mindful eating*, however, takes on particular relevance from as early as childhood in the context of exchanges, related to nutrition, between children and caregivers. Hirschmann and Zaphiropoulos (2012) emphasize the importance of "on demand" nutrition, based on three steps (eating when one is hungry, eating foods one feels the need for, stopping when one feels full) which, in the case of children, are often mediated by the intervention of the adult who establishes, in a certain sense, what are the "right" foods at a certain time of the day and of developmental stage, thus transforming an internal self-regulation process in one governed by external factors. The role of parents, according to the authors, should be to *promote awareness in children of internal stimuli related to hunger and satiety*. In other words, it is a process in which the non-judgemental attitude of parents allows the child to acquire self-regulating abilities.

A *mindful-oriented* attitude, in parent–child relationships, can promote the breakdown of dysfunctional patterns and enable greater attunement by parents (Gambrel & Keeling 2010; Siegel 2007; Wachs & Cordoba 2007). The concept of *mindful parenting* extends that of mindfulness in describing the ability of parents to fully attentively listen to the child, to accept themselves and the child in a non-judgemental way, to be aware of the emotions of both, to self-regulate in the parental relationship and experience compassion[9] for themselves and their child.

The ability to listen with full attention does not only concern attention to what is being said; rather it implies the ability to listen by activating a focused attention that enables one to grasp elements of communication that go beyond what is being said. Its origins are traceable in the early exchanges in which the crying or the behaviours of the child act as distress signals, inducing the parent's response through a process of deep emotional attunement and of construction of the internal representation of the child. Later, when the child is older, the *mindful* parent will be able to grasp not only what the child says but also the tone of voice, the facial expression and other elements, so as to be able to deeply grasp the emotional state of the child. This process seems to be clearly connected to the ability to accept oneself and the child in a non-judgemental manner, which does not mean taking on a defeatist attitude, but accepting what is happening in the present moment with awareness and attention so as to reach a greater level of understanding. This implies, for example, the possibility of also accepting the critical aspects of parenthood, such as the physiological aspects of conflict of the parent–child relationship. *Mindful* parents will also be able to recognize their own emotions and those of their child, managing to regulate themselves in the relational context and thus decreasing their reactivity. The final characteristic of *mindful parenting*, that is the ability to feel compassion for oneself and for one's own child, concerns the possibility of experiencing an empathic concern for the latter but also for oneself, taking on a less severe position towards one's own efforts as a parent.

Duncan, Coatsworth and Greenberg (2009) underline the importance of *mindful parenting* in the dynamic process of the relationship between parents and adolescents in which remarkable changes can be observed, although the quality of the relationship might remain fairly stable. In the transition to adolescence, parents and children experience less physical closeness, the intensification of conflict and the demand for greater autonomy. Parents could be activated by what their children say or do, experiencing emotional and behavioural reactions that could also lead to hard interventions in terms of discipline. Consequently, adolescents who, from a developmental point of view, experience greater difficulty in managing negative emotions could react strongly, thus feeding a circle of negative emotions (what in systemic terms is referred to as *symmetrical escalation*). *Mindful parenting* could clearly be considered a protective factor with respect to the relationship and to the fulfilling of the developmental tasks of adolescence.

Although *mindfulness* could be considered a key factor with respect to the functional adaptation of parents and children, its integration into a more complex model that takes into account other factors that influence family development and functioning is fundamental to being able to reach a fuller understanding of the phenomenon itself and the results of a possible intervention. Harnett and Dawe (2013) highlight how *mindfulness*-based interventions can be more functionally considered as possible underlying strategies for achieving positive outcomes in the relationship with children and their families rather than as interventions in and of themselves. Changes with respect to the level of *mindfulness* can in fact be looked at as mediators and moderators of change in different areas of family functioning. The integrated model proposed by the Authors aims to promote positive outcomes in child development in different areas of functioning and over time by identifying proximal and more distal family functioning areas, such as the quality of the parent–child relationship, with specific reference to the parents' emotional availability and the way they behave with respect to their role, their values as parents and their expectations of the child as factors capable of influencing the educational choices made by the parents, on the levels of monitoring of the child and the importance of family routines.

Although there is no intervention based on *mindfulness* specifically designed for clinical work with families, the fundamental dimensions of *mindful parenting* seem to correspond to possible work objectives and, at the same time, to evaluation tools, in line with the idea that a relational (or structural) change might bring about a deeper (intrapsychic) change, activated in the therapeutic space and through the analysis of what happens in the session (present moment). What we intend to highlight, in this chapter, is the opportunity to insert, within family therapy, elements that belong to different theoretical frameworks, following the idea that there are multiple "entry points" through which to approach relational dynamics (Sameroff 2004).

The following clinical vignette therefore represents an attempt to work on family dynamics in a case of food selectivity in pre-adolescence, using some *mindful parenting* concepts as activators and promoters of change.

4. A clinical case

The therapist receives a telephone call from Ms A explaining that she received her contact from her GP, worried about the feeding behaviour of Sandro, Ms

A's 11-year-old eldest son. She in fact says her son eats little in terms of quantity and is rather selective with respect to the variety of foods, limiting his diet to plain pasta and parmesan cheese. Meat is absent, as is fruit, while vegetables and pulses are eaten only if completely blended and reduced "to almost the consistency of baby food". On the other hand, Sandro would be happy eating only chocolate and pre-packaged snacks that his parents partly tend to limit. Ms A says she is "exasperated" by her son's behaviour but does not know "absolutely what to do … whether to force him or let him go on like this".

A first interview session with the whole family (mother, father, Sandro and his sister Marta, aged 8) is suggested, to discuss the family context in which the symptom manifested itself, to understand its probable function within it, and to analyse the reasons behind their request for therapeutic help. Often, in fact, the family's implicit request is to modify the "designated patient", thinking this may restore the conditions preceding the onset of symptoms, in an attempt to defend family homeostasis.

On the day of the session the whole family arrives on time at the therapist's study. They are all well presented and well behaved, but Sandro's appearance seems to contradict his relational manners. He is a tiny boy, appearing younger than his 11 years, who, however, greets the therapist by shaking her hand like a tiny adult. When they enter the room, the parents invite Sandro to sit between them while Marta positions herself outside, next to her father. At first glance, Sandro and Marta appear quite different: the former is thin with a rather pale face and a somewhat sad expression, while the latter seems to be slightly overweight, with an open and smiling expression.

The mother works as an employee and has decided to only work part time since the birth of her children, while the father is a freelancer, very busy with work, so much so that he spends most of his time away from home, often even past dinner time. The families of origin of both parents are described as traditional ones, with mothers dedicated to the family and the home, and fathers focused on working. Sandro's parents met when they were 25 through mutual friends and they got married after nine years of relationship, sharing the idea of building a family.

The parents express deep concern because Sandro refuses to eat most of the foods that he is offered. Both parents underline the rigidity of this eating behaviour and the refusal to eat if he is presented with the "wrong" foods, describing Sandro as a child who has always been "picky" and unwilling to try new foods. Food selectivity seems to have worsened between the end of primary school and the beginning of middle school, a passage apparently experienced without difficulties. Sandro himself says that he likes going to school, where he gets good – often excellent – grades even though, because of "all the homework I have to do, I often have to give up seeing my friends, but it doesn't matter". Marta also does well in school, though she admits to preferring extra-curricular activities.

The mother describes how mealtimes, especially lunchtime, have become filled with conflict. Sandro, from the beginning of middle school, has lunch at home, alone with his mother; in the experience of both, it seems that those moments follow an actual script, with the mother who initially tries to suggest foods that are different from his preferred ones, Sandro opposes this, to the point of totally refusing to eat, activating the angry reaction of the mother who, however, ends up giving up for fear that her son will not take in the right amount of calories. The father, on the other hand, is not worried by this aspect because he is aware that the child tends to compensate by eating chocolate or other snacks; he also underlines that when all the family gathers for mealtime, there seems to be less conflict: the mother is less insistent on trying to make Sandro eat different foods and seems more able to tolerate his protests, also because the father often interrupts the exchanges between mother and child, reassuring his wife that the important thing is that "the child eats something" and that mealtimes "does not turn into a war".

Both parents stress that "apart from conflicts regarding food" there are no other reasons for arguing in the family. Sandro seems to have always fully satisfied the expectations of his parents, proving to be attentive and disciplined both at home and at school. Up until the end of primary school, as his father says, "he was perfect".

The explicit request formulated by the parents, to which Sandro seems to adhere only formally, is focused on food and the possibility of modifying his eating behaviour towards a decrease in restriction. Marta is the only member asking for help "not to quarrel", thus shifting attention, albeit unconsciously, from the concrete aspect of food and nutrition to the relational dimension that underlies it.

A biweekly therapeutic intervention is suggested to the family and is accepted by all members. Three months after the start of treatment, a further suggestion is made, to alternate family sessions, with all four members, with couple sessions, aimed at working with the mother and father on parenting and marital issues.

During the sessions, certain particularly relevant aspects emerge. Firstly, Sandro was breastfed until he was one, notwithstanding having started weaning around the age of five months with no particular difficulty for the child, but with a considerable level of concern for the mother who feared introducing new foods because potentially unwelcome or difficult to swallow. Although Sandro was curious, experimenting with new flavours and textures was strictly regulated by the mother who gave directions/rules on how and what was right to eat. Ms A, for example, says that she continued to spoon-feed her son for a long time to be able to check the amount of food the child put in his mouth and whether he swallowed it without difficulty. The husband adds that it was difficult for Sandro to even be able to eat a biscuit by himself, without this activating maternal anxiety and without the mother resorting to breaking it up into small pieces, which she did for most of the foods that, according to her, could represent a potential danger for the child. This happened even though Sandro's teeth had come out and the child was showing a certain "voracity" in trying to bite food. The mother remembers being almost frightened by this behaviour, that made her child look like a "tiny predator". The transition from breastfeeding to solid food intake represents for the child the opportunity to experience a certain amount of aggression necessary to bite and chew, to some extent to destroy the food that is coming from the outside, offered by the mother. The mother's discomfort when witnessing Sandro's voracity/aggression seems to have been solved, unconsciously, through worrying that the child might "choke" and the subsequent adoption of a hyper-controlling behaviour that involved breaking up food and thus avoiding chewing. The mother's ability to tolerate her son's aggressive attack during the early stages seems to have transformed, in the current relationship, where no conflict is reported in relation to Sandro's developmental phase, in which aggression is functional to being able to distance oneself from the parents' model and to acquire one's own identity.

Sandro's father had never managed to enter, as a "third", in the symbiotic relationship between Sandro and his mother, activating his function as mediator in the relationship with the outside world and as support with regard to his wife's emotion regulation. Marta, unlike her brother, seems to have had a more linear development, transitioning from breastfeeding to weaning without difficulties and with a progressive but constant replacement of milk with solid foods.

After a few sessions, the presence of sleep difficulties also emerges, to address which, from an early age, Sandro has needed the closeness of one of his parents. The processes related to sleep and nutrition appear to be dysregulated and Sandro continues to seek a regulation for them through his parents, as if he were a young infant. The positions taken by family members during the first session and for a long time after the start of treatment, with Sandro between and very close to his parents and Marta close to her father, but projected outside, seem to reflect what could be defined as a difficulty in exploration, intended as a consequence of early interactions characterized by insecurity and poor responsiveness by the caregiver.

This arrangement also seems to have a correspondence in terms of interpersonal relationships: Sandro appears closed and selective in his relationship with peers, preferring to engage in activities with his family and maintaining symbiotic relationships. During sessions, he often seeks his mother's gaze, he touches her, receiving affectionate gestures in return, such as fixing his hair or shirt or even apparently automatic gestures, such as tying his shoes up without anyone, including Sandro, being surprised by this. If we think of a family as a structure, that is, as "a network of functional needs that organize the way in which the members of a family system interact" (Malagoli Togliatti & Cotugno 1996, p. 223), Sandro's position within his family appears functional on the one hand to the maintenance of a fusional mother–child relationship and on the other to the role of mediator with respect to the couple. Thus, the family seems to be organized in subsystems, such as mother–Sandro, father–Marta and mother–Sandro–father, that seem to be well represented in the sessions through the way in which the family members physically position themselves.

Starting, in fact, from a concrete change of spatial disposition, with the therapist asking Sandro to be moved between the father and the sister, so as to avoid his being next to the mother and between the parents, it was possible to let the family experience, in the *here* and *now*, a new configuration that enabled work on the subsystems, "revealing the identities of the family members" (Minuchin, Reiter, & Borda 2013) and working on the subjective experiences and the representational aspects brought by each member. The therapist must, however, be mindful of the fact that the family system tends to maintain homeostasis and such a movement could be seen as dangerous precisely because it threatens the balance of the system and forces it towards a redefinition of its boundaries, that is, of the rules that determine *who participates and how*. It is essential that the therapist joins the family through an attitude of curiosity and empathy so as to be able to question the certainties of the family and promote change by introducing a new, non-judgemental perspective, also through the use of humour and metaphors.

Working with Sandro's family, a choice was made to work on the *here* and *now*, focusing initially on the present moment relating to exchanges like that centred on the tying up of Sandro's shoes, investigating the underlying emotional state of each member and interrupting the automatism of a gesture "done without thinking", as the mother often said. These exchanges allow the therapist to work on a theme that, while connected to the problem brought into therapy, is not explicit, shifting, for example, attention from food to autonomy as a central element of growth and development of both Sandro and the entire family. It is possible to investigate what the experience is for all members with respect to what happens during the session, revealing, in the case of Sandro's family, the ambivalence of the mother, but also of the child, towards the separation process connected to development, well represented by the desire that Sandro "would eat like us adults" while remaining dependent in relation to other dimensions of autonomy.

Asking "Why do you tie Sandro's shoes up?" also revealed the mother's hypervigilance with respect to her behaviour as a parent, often characterized by the fear of not being adequate and making mistakes that would cause her son to reject her, according to a rather naive and simplistic interpretation of the equation between nutrition and maternal figure ("doctor, it is known that food represents the mother so Sandro has a problem with me, I'm obviously at fault"). It seems clear that the mother constantly judges herself and the relationship, rather than reflecting on what functional needs might lie behind the symptom.

The father's emphasizing of the frequency of such behaviours and of his not agreeing with them enabled the introduction of a new variable, namely his being peripheral, well represented by the phrase "I am never there, what could I do to help them?" By suggesting to the family that they should observe what happens without judgement but promoting an awareness of the mental and emotional state of each member, one also promotes a process of deconstruction and restructuring of the family organization and a redefinition of the symptomatic aspects, i.e., a new interpretation of the factors that determined the disorder according to a circular causality. The therapist thus promotes a non-judgemental acceptance of the symptomatic manifestations by suggesting the family could reinterpret them as functional elements for communicating something that would otherwise be unspeakable, which concerns the entire family and not the individual, and freeing the parents from feeling guilty for causing them; for example, the mother's sense of inadequacy, connected to her past history but also to the poor support she experienced in her relationship with her husband; the latter's inability to enter the mother–child relationship breaking its symbiosis but also his feeling of exclusion at the birth of his first child.

Such passages were possible through what, in *mindful parenting*, is defined as non-judgemental acceptance of oneself in one's own parental role. The adoption of this perspective can lead to a reduction in conflict that is often amplified by the parent's unconscious need to repair or erase the error that led to the disorder: understanding what happened in the past by reflecting on the underlying intrapsychic and relational emotional aspects enables the adoption of an attitude that is on one hand more compassionate and on the other more open to change.

The symptom brought into therapy becomes an opportunity to reflect on the rigidity of family functioning, searching for the critical event that triggered the dysfunctional adjustments. The acceptance of this perspective, introduced by the therapist, enables a reinterpretation of the entire family history and of the subjective experiences of the individual members. It was thus possible to go back to the birth of Sandro, following which the mother experienced an excessive burden of responsibility with respect to the growth of her child, trying to be the perfect mother instead of a "sufficiently good" mother (Winnicott 1971). The frequent absence of her husband, busy with work and not very able to support his wife in a functional way with respect to parenthood, left his wife alone with her concern of not being adequate enough and of being potentially harmful, for example proposing solid foods that are difficult to swallow, but also alone in facing the aggressiveness of her child, intended as a necessary element for the acquisition of greater autonomy and for the affirmation of his identity.

Sandro's food selectivity was thus redefined as the emerging, visible aspect of a larger structure. The eating symptom, therefore, is not the only element on which to focus attention but can be redefined as the piece of a puzzle the meaning of which becomes clear only once it is completed, in the union of all pieces. In therapy, it was thus possible to connect the emerging symptom to the difficulty in falling asleep, to the relational selectivity but also to the different management of food by Marta who "eats everything", thus avoiding conflict with her parents but also their excessive attention, and managing in this way to break away with less difficulty. The puzzle thus composed seems to show a difficulty for the family in facing a transition to the developmental phase that follows early childhood.

Verification and analysis of this hypothesis (Selvini Palazzoli, Boscolo, Cecchin, & Prata 1980) was explored in therapy by asking Sandro to move and sit next to his sister, creating a specific *present moment*[10] aimed at investigating the emotions and the states of mind of each with respect to a new distance–closeness balance. Sandro, in saying "I kind of like it, but I also kind of don't like it", was able to express his own ambivalence with respect to the exasperated search for physical and emotional proximity with his mother, an ambivalence well expressed by the eating symptom that on one side relates to the permanence of more infantile aspects and on the other to the emergence of functional opposition with respect to the activation of a process of autonomization and disengagement from the parents.

The activation of the father, particularly through the work on the parental subsystem during the couple sessions, allowed Mr A to understand the wife's point of view, becoming an effective provider of support for her, and to take on the role of promoter and facilitator of his children's exploration.

Gradually, Sandro started to introduce new foods but, above all, he began to experiment with a greater differentiation from his parental figures and from the mother in particular, investing more on his relationship with peers and starting to search for the "right distance" from his parental figures.

This passage is evidenced by the need to define one's own belonging to the group of peers, that leads pre-adolescents to compare themselves with the *other*, taking into consideration, sometimes acquiring, the *other*'s behaviours not only as a functional strategy to be accepted but, above all, as a way to experiment with modalities that differ from one's own. The presence of siblings in therapy enables work on these aspects, starting from the different behavioural strategies, activating a reciprocal process of reflection and "learning".

Not dwelling on the concrete aspects related to food, not providing the family with behavioural indications with respect to the management of eating, but using what happens *around food* to broaden the view on the entire system enables the creation of space to activate a change. Although questioning the certainties of the family initially activates their resistances, as they feel their homeostatic balance threatened, the therapist's ability to explore alternatives and use the content of communications to understand the process of family dynamics, uncovering the identity of the members and accompanying the family in the change of its structural organization, enables the promotion of a dialogue between what happens externally, in the dimension of reality, and what happens on the subjective experiential level. This brings about a greater awareness and acceptance of the emotions experienced by each of the members; the emotional aspects can thus be mentalized and not acted out through the symptom.

5. Conclusions

Family-based interventions require a constant oscillation between relational and individual aspects, interactional exchanges and intrapsychic and representational dimensions. It could be said that they represent a clinical context in which to *naturally* experiment with the integration of constructs and models relating to different theoretical frameworks.

The intervention of the therapist as an element of the system enables a focus on family organization and, at the same time, the introduction of elements related to the processes of mentalization and *mindfulness*, facilitating the acquisition by the family of a new approach to understand the critical, normative and paranormative events, which denote its life cycle.

The construct of *mindfulness* can be found within different interventions such as DBT (Linehan 1987), stress reduction interventions often used in medicine (MBSR – *mindfulness-based stress reduction*; Tacón, Caldera, & Ronaghan 2004) from which a couple-focused programme was derived (MBRE – *mindfulness-based relationship enhancement*; Carson, Carson, Gil, & Baucom 2006), and interventions focused on parenting (*mindful parenting*).

Cohen-Katz (2004) suggested the possibility of evaluating the effect of MBSR interventions on the entire family system, emphasizing the change in the individual as an activator of new possible family configurations or, to put it in other terms, as "disturber" of family homeostasis. The different models of family therapy place emphasis on the *here* and *now* and this aspect can be integrated with an attention to the *present moment* on which *mindfulness*-based interventions are focused. Dwelling on the *present moment* in therapy allows the patient, each of the members of the family, to experience a new awareness and a non-judgemental acceptance of the self and the other. These aspects can take on particular importance during the course of treatment, not so much as final objectives or solutions of the difficulty brought into therapy by the family but as tools through which to start exploring ever more complex dimensions regarding the family and the individual history of each member, the meaning of the symptom within the family and the possible developmental trajectories, using what happens in the *here* and *now* of the therapy to identify communication and relationship models (Watzlawick & Beavin 1967). In therapeutic work with families of pre-adolescent individuals with an eating disorder, the possibility of adopting a deeply non-judgemental point of view of oneself and the other through a *mindful-oriented* approach enables the start of an exploration of the meaning of the symptom within the family rather than seeking its extinction through defensive behaviours that tend to deny its relational value and that hinder change. The promotion of a compassionate attitude in the context of family relationships seems to be a protective factor with respect to the ability of the entire family to face the developmental tasks of each phase of the family's life cycle and, in particular, the beginning of pre-adolescence for the children, which brings about a series of challenges regarding the processes of separation–identification and a deep re-structuring of roles.

Highlights

- Middle childhood, referring to children between 7 and 12 years of age, highlights the children's tendency to continue searching for available attachment figures, while recognizing the decreasingly exclusive value of this relationship.
- Attachment security continues to act as a functional factor for exploration which, in this specific period of development, can be understood in a broad sense as the possibility of "exploring" new relationships and the emotions associated with physical, cognitive and social changes.
- Food selectivity is often already present in early childhood and is distinguished from neophobias because it concerns the refusal of foods that are familiar to the child. These problems, often referred to as *picky or fussy eating*, are more frequent in preschool age, with a peak incidence at the age of six, and can last up to the age of 11 with similar characteristics in childhood and pre-adolescence.
- Through exploration of the family system and of its subsystems it is possible to understand the role of each member with respect to the dysfunctional, symptomatic model brought into therapy, thus shifting the focus from the designated patient to the system as a whole.
- The *mentalization-based treatment for families* promotes awareness of the impact of one's own thoughts, feelings and actions on the other, the ability to take on a confident, humble and playful attitude, the belief that change is possible, the acceptance of responsibility, as well as forgiveness, intended as the ability to reinterpret other individuals' actions on the basis of an understanding and acceptance of their mental states.
- The clinician can activate reflection on these aspects through *curiosity*, understood as a means that can "challenge" the family's certainties that hinder change, explore alternatives and use the content to understand the process, highlighting the *circularity*, that is the concatenation of a series of family system states, through the exploration of the subjective experiences of each member of the family.
- Although there is no intervention based on *mindfulness* specifically designed for clinical work with families, the fundamental dimensions of *mindful parenting* seem to correspond to possible work objectives and, at the same time, to evaluation tools, in line with the idea that a relational (or structural) change might bring about a deeper (intrapsychic) change,

activated in the therapeutic space and through the analysis of what happens in the session (present moment).

Notes

1 This process also appears to be related to sensitive, responsive and accepting parenting practices, to the (secure) mental state of the parent and to the family environment. The children of disengaged or enmeshed families have lower levels of security than children of cohesive and adequate families (Davies, Cummings, & Winter 2004).

2 What appears to be relevant, in terms of differential diagnosis with respect to other food-related disorders, is the absence of concerns with body weight, which is often in line with what is identified by growth curves, and of difficulties in ingesting food for fear of vomiting and choking.

3 Recent publications have highlighted the role of breastfeeding as an "appetite regulator" (Li, Fein, & Grummer-Strawn 2010) as it leads the mother to focus her attention on the child's hunger and satiety signals rather than on the amount of milk offered; this mechanism would allow a decrease in the mother's tendency to exercise control in favour of a more responsive attitude towards the child (de Campora, Giromini, Larciprete, Li Volsi, & Zavattini 2014; de Campora, D'Onofrio, & Zavattini 2014).

4 Relationship rules affect mutual behaviours of family members in a circular dynamic and must be flexible to be able to adapt to changes, especially in the passage between different life-cycle phases. The rigidity of these rules could lead to a developmental block, which crystallizes the system into its previous equilibrium and increases the risk that the suffering of the entire family becomes translated into the symptomatic behaviour of a single individual.

5 According to Bowen (1979), the process of differentiation contrasts the attempt to maintain the undifferentiated *family Ego* mass, that is "a *conglomerate emotional oneness* where one cannot distinguish where the one's self begins and where that of the other ends" (Andolfi 2002, p. 33).

6 Literature presents follow-up studies (Herscovici & Bay 1996; Martin 1985; Mayer 1994; Minuchin, Rosman, & Baker 1978) and randomized clinical trials (Eisler et al. 2000; le Grange, Eisler, Dare, & Russell 1992; Robin et al. 1999) where different forms of family therapy were compared.

7 The FBT includes three phases, the first of which is focused on the behavioural aspects (reduction of food intake, compensation behaviours) and sees the involvement of parents in the child's "re-nutrition" and weight recovery. Having achieved this objective, the second and third phases shift the focus of the intervention on the gradual acquisition of greater autonomy on the part of the children initially with respect to their own eating and, subsequently, through the exploration of the other areas of functioning (scholastic, social, family related, etc.).

8 It is an intervention model stemming from a cognitive-behavioural perspective, initially developed for the treatment of patients with severe suicidal risk and later applied to patients with borderline personality disorder; it includes a group intervention aimed at developing specific skills, an individual intervention and telephone coaching. The specific skills developed through DBT concern *mindfulness,* tolerance of suffering, interpersonal efficacy and emotion regulation.

9 According to Gilbert (2005), compassion is defined by six components, or "attributes": caring for others, sensitivity to suffering, active participation (sympathy), empathy, tolerance to suffering and non-judgemental attitude. Sensitivity and

tolerance to suffering are distinct because the former implies the ability to feel, recognize and distinguish one's own needs and discomforts from those of the other, while the latter refers to the ability to contain and tolerate emotional intensity. Similarly, active participation and empathy differ because the second involves cognitive understanding of others, the ability to take their point of view, and not only the ability to be emotionally involved.

10 With this expression, we refer to the definition of "present moment" used in the context of *mindfulness*.

Chapter 7

Bulimia and adolescence

Mojgan Khademi and Heidi Miller Brunetto

I. Bulimia and adolescence: theoretical overview

Core features of bulimia are binge eating followed by inappropriate compensatory behaviors such as self-induced vomiting, laxative or diuretic misuse, fasting and excessive exercise. The patient experiences a loss of control during the overeating, followed by guilt and remorse (Le Grange & Schmidt, 2005). These features most commonly emerge in mid-adolescence and the observed lifetime prevalence estimates for all forms of eating disorder (ED) are similar to those reported for US adults (Swanson, Crow, Le Grange, Swendsen, & Merikangas, 2011). Dieting, which starts early among female adolescents, is considered the most important predictor of new eating disorders among them, along with comorbid psychiatric problems (Patton, Selzer, Coffey, Carlin, & Wolfe, 1999).

Female socialization is considered a major risk factor in bulimia among adolescents, centered on the role of beauty in the female sex-role stereotype, along with biological, psychological and family influences. There is growing recognition that symptom-focused treatments do not fully address this complex disorder (Thompson-Brenner, Weingeroff, & Westen, 2009) and growing consensus that patients with ED have interpersonal problems (Hartmann, Zeeck, & Barrett, 2010), including adolescents (Patton et al., 1999). This warrants an integrated approach that addresses the complexity of the problem among adolescents.

Bulimia has been explained as a purely cognitive psychopathology (Fairburn, 2008), as well as one related to core failures during the separation/individuation phase (Sugarman & Kurash, 1982), a reflection of ego deficits related to regulation of intolerable internal states (Casper, 1983), a compromise formation between impulse and prohibition, a means of regulating affective, as well as protection of self against fragmentation (Yarock, 1993). The binge/purge cycle has been considered a re-enactment of experiencing the mother as forcing herself and her wishes upon the young girl, which can only be dealt with by vomiting out (Farrell, 2001). In addition, their typical oppositionality is believed to represent an attempt to bolster their sense of self (de Groot & Rodin, 1994).

According to Cognitive Behavioral Theory (CBT), all forms of ED, including bulimia "share a distinctive core psychopathology that is cognitive in nature" expressed in a variety of ways such as eating habits. Dysfunctional schemes for self-evaluation are seen as responsible for most of the patients' difficulties, although binge eating is understood primarily as a byproduct of restrictive dieting (Fairburn, 2008).

From a psychodynamic perspective, EDs result from gender-specific conflicts expressed through the body, i.e., the body is used, instead of words, to express conflicts around dependence and sexuality. Similar to CBT, the body is believed to take on an excessively central role for the continuity of the sense of self with physical attributes such as weight reflecting states of well-being, control and self-worth. CBT considers all ED patients as failing to connect their own behaviors to day-to-day events and negative moods (Fairburn, 2008). Psychodynamic perspective expands this idea to include them failing to understand their day-to-day behaviors and negative mood in relation to mental states, such as thoughts or feelings – referred to as mentalization (Fonagy & Target, 2000). This capacity for mentalization correlates with attachment security and empirical investigations have shown that individuals with ED tend to be insecurely attached (Troisi, Massaroni, & Cuzzolaro, 2005) and show impairments in mentalization (Skarderud, 2007; Ward, Ramsay, Turnbull, Benedettini, & Treasure, 2000), which predict body dissatisfaction (Troisi et al. 2006). Similarly, among normal pre-adolescent girls, insecure attachment has been found to correlate with poor mentalization and higher risk of developing an ED (Cate, Khademi, Judd, & Miller, 2013).

2. The clinical approach

Cognitive Behavioral Therapy (CBT) has been adapted for treatment of bulimia with success in adults (NICE, 2004) and adolescents (Fairburn, 2008). Offering alternative treatments is suggested, however, when patients fail to improve substantially or experience a setback (Fairburn, 2008). Similarly, CBT Guided Self-Care was found to be superior to family therapy with bulimic adolescents, due to its specific focus on bingeing as a specific problem (Schmidt et al., 2007).

An integrated psychodynamic treatment of bulimia considers the theoretical contributions of both CBT and psychodynamic approaches. The strategy underpinning CBT is to construct a set of hypotheses that maintain the ED psychopathology in order to identify features to be targeted in treatment (Fairburn, 2008). An integrated psychodynamic approach maintains this idea, but includes a broader range of hypotheses to be considered, i.e. bulimic symptoms not only involve cognitive distortions, but are also designed to deny, anesthetize or discharge unwanted internal states that precede, coincide with, or follow interpersonal exchanges (Moreno, 1998). Difficulties with self-awareness, self-acceptance, self-expression (Aranson, 1993), separation, autonomy (Patton, 1992), dependence (Bornstein & Greenberg, 1991) and discriminating emotional responses from bodily ones (Herkov, Greer, Blau, McGuire, & Eaker, 1994) are considered relevant to their symptoms. Furthermore, interpretations and the therapeutic relationship are considered central in the treatment of bulimia and binge eating disorders (William, 1997; Zerbe, 2001).

An integrated psychodynamic approach incorporates techniques from both approaches, but emphasizes the use of the therapeutic relationship. CBT focuses on developing strategies to eat regularly and appropriately, to cope with specific symptoms and to address irrational thoughts and behaviors using explicit advice and self-monitoring homework. Both approaches consider the establishment of a therapeutic relationship important. The psychodynamic approach recognized that the very process of "taking things in has gone wrong" (Farrell, 2001, p. 61) for these patients, which requires paying close attention to the therapeutic relationship, including identifying unconscious conflicts, interpersonal patterns, unacceptable feelings (especially anger) in general, as well as in the transference.

A combined CBT and psychodynamic approach has been suggested for treatment in general when chronic characterological issues interfere with the success of traditional CBT approaches (Young, Kolosko, & Weishaar, 2003). Anxiety and depressive symptoms, as well as chronic comorbid disorders are considered common among ED patients (Fairburn, 2008; Kaye, Bulik, Thornton, Barbarich, & Masters, 2004) and experienced clinicians report frequent comorbidity (substance abuse; depression; anxiety) and use of a combination of treatment strategies with ED patients (Thompson-Brenner & Westen, 2005). There is empirical evidence that psychodynamically oriented short-term (20–40 sessions) psychotherapy that integrates behavioral principles related to ED is as equally effective as CBT (Murphy, Russell, & Waller, 2005).

An integrated psychodynamic approach also reflects findings that countertransference is an important factor in treatment of EDs (Satir, Thompson-Brenner, Boisseau, & Crisafulli, 2009) since feelings of social incompetence, low self-esteem and a lack of perceived personal effectiveness are common (Hartmann et al., 2010). The bulimic adolescent has spent her life avoiding being known, which is manifested as attempts to control the therapist and preventing an emotional connection (Farrell, 2001).

A thorough assessment of symptoms and interpersonal functioning is essential to an integrated psychodynamic approach. In addition, the therapist must focus on assessing the adolescent's history regarding weight with attention to their early body-esteem (Killen et al. 1994), negative experiences with caregivers (Perkins et al., 2005; Winn et al., 2007), as well as family history of EDs (Strober, Lampert, Morell, Burroughs, & Jacobs, 1990), which are considered risk factors. Furthermore, affect and self-esteem regulation as well intimate relationships – romantic and otherwise – should be explored (Costin, 2006). Patients with ED feel misunderstood and being cumulatively misunderstood is traumatic. They expect the therapist to be a misunderstanding mother and adapt to this by withdrawing or rushing from one topic to the next – becoming apparently misunderstandable (Farrell, 2001).

An integrated psychodynamic approach addresses not only symptoms, but especially relevant variables of motivation, insight and resistance, while it emphasizes the importance of understanding the emotional reactions of both the patient and the therapist (Murphy et al., 2005). Interpretations and the therapeutic relationship are central since words are as problematic as their relationship to food (Farrell, 2001). This requires the therapist to use words, especially to demonstrate one's authenticity and to be the antithesis of the ED patient, i.e. flexible, creative, genuine and willing to take risks by talking about what is happening in the room. Working with the countertransference is recommended as "the way" to work with these patients, allowing the patient to use the therapist as an intermediate object (Farrell, 2001).

The development of a working alliance is followed by formulation of hypotheses about the underlying focal conflicts and their relation to bulimia. Teaching the patient to self-monitor, using an Emotional State/Binge/Purge Diary to connect external events, feelings and behaviors is adapted from CBT. The emphasis is on understanding their behaviors, as opposed to altering them, however, and to illuminate conflicts and compromise formations. As they learn about their own responses, they can gain a greater sense of agency (Murphy et al., 2005) leading to increased interest in and motivation for behavioral change. Consultation with a nutritionist or medical professionals is utilized to offer guidance regarding behavioral change. In short, helping ED patients understand their own minds and putting their previously somaticized reactions into words, with a therapist brave enough to be authentic in any given moment, are essential to treatment.

3. Case discussion

Sophia was lovely, by every account. Anxious, especially when she talked about feeling out of control bingeing on cereal and peanut butter late at night, or exercising endlessly the following morning. Tall and thin, she was attractive, pleasant and easy to like. But she led an isolated life, dominated by her exercise regimen, undergraduate studies and more recently anxiety of applying to law school. The fact that her worsening symptoms of anxiety and eating disorder had begun to interfere with her academic aspirations had finally led her to seek help.

Sophia's behavior seemed mysterious and inexplicable to her, except for the fact that somehow it made her feel better – if only for a moment. She puzzled over her good and bad days, her inability to stop eating or exercising, and was unable to connect them with any particular internal reaction or external event. This failure to mentalize left her either overwhelmed or worried about inexplicably becoming overwhelmed.

Sophia's personal history shed some light on her insecure attachment and mentalization deficits, which correspond with body dissatisfaction (Troisi et al. 2006). She also reported her family to have paid close attention to weight and appearance (Senra, Sanchez-Cao, Seoane & Leung, 2006). As a shy child in an otherwise loud and turbulent family, with a father prone to temper tantrums, a mother who preferred to look the other way, and older siblings who created conflict and overshadowed her, Sophia kept everything to herself and resorted to fantasy to cope. She experienced her parents as either ignoring her or putting pressure on her to perform athletically and academically, on which she herself focused in order to escape and to establish a sense of efficacy. Her feelings, left unexplored and non-verbalized left her unable to make sense of her experiences.

The issues that Sophia seemed unable to make psychological sense of were numerous. For example, she could only verbalize that she had felt "sick to her stomach" after a session in which we eventually discovered she had been angry with me. Also, her insecure attachment style had serious transference implications as she was quick to assume that she was one minor infraction (e.g. being late) away from being kicked out of treatment.

Sophia's conflicts were often activated within interpersonal relationships. Her feelings of social incompetence and low self-esteem caused her to feel personally ineffective and unable to get what she wanted from others. It was easy to see the worry she had about actually experiencing the loneliness that awaited her at the end of the day. This feeling alone and uncared for was a major interpersonal theme for Sophia. In friendships, Sophia was guarded and had trouble feeling close. Romantic relationships were devalued and avoided, since she expected to feel disappointed and foolish. When a male classmate showed some interest in her, she was panicked: "What if I decide I like him and tomorrow he won't be there!" With me, she feared that needing me would cause me to disappear.

A closer look at the connection between her symptoms and her interpersonal relationships was warranted. She was certainly likable, as evidenced by my positive countertransference, but her inability to interact in a manner that was genuine and reflected her feelings and opinions caused her to easily feel disappointed and to withdraw. For example, she felt "used" as a sounding board for friends with whom she could not effectively assert herself. Similarly, she felt devastated and betrayed when friends, not grasping the extreme importance of Sophia's most minor self-disclosures, shared minor details about her family with one another. Hurt and tearful, Sophia could not see how the urgency of keeping everything inside, had created her reaction.

Once the therapeutic alliance was established – albeit regularly monitored – I focused on suggesting hypotheses to connect her symptoms, life events and feelings based on what she wrote in the emotional state/binge/purge diary. In addition to her learning to self-monitor, the diary allowed us to make sense of her reactions. This helped illuminate her conflicts around many interpersonal issues including competition with friends, separation from her family and sexuality. For example, when she binged after her friend flirted with a man that Sophia had admired from afar, the diary allowed us to identify and put into words the unacceptable feelings she had tried to escape through action – envy, competition and rage.

Systematically verbalizing what was happening in our relationship was an essential part of treatment. Once, in response to Sophia's complaint about her friends "talking at" her, I pointed out how a similar thing could have happened with us. She seemed confused by my statement, so as matter of factly as I could, I described her subtle, non-verbal signals (i.e. looking away and seeming disinterested, not listening) that I had observed at times when I seemed to have talked a bit too long for her liking. Up to this point, I had merely reacted behaviorally (i.e. I had stopped talking and redirected the conversation to her) and had allowed her to communicate by impact (Casement, 1991). I framed my observations in terms of what her friends may miss, which could lead to her feeling used. She confessed to some awareness that at times she had stopped listening to what I was saying, but was surprised that I had noticed this, as though she expected to be invisible. After this encounter, we both seemed to be freer to think and feel. I recognized the projective identification process, i.e. how she had helped me experientially know how she had been treated as a child (King, 1978) and how, in the absence of actual intimacy, I had felt insecure in her attachment to me and had become overly compliant, just as she had with her mother. As she explored our interactions more freely, she considered that perhaps her friends were not as uncaring as she imagined and wondered about her contribution to the shortcomings of her relationships. We could then focus on thoughts and fantasies that interfered with her speaking her mind (e.g. not knowing how she felt; fear of losing control if she put her feelings into words, and of course the fear of rejection if others knew how she felt). Accustomed to living an unauthentic life, and expecting all others to do the same, she seemed amazed and excited about comments that reflected my willingness to talk about her, myself and our reactions to each other. This led to true insight, i.e. one derived from affect-laden experiences with the therapist, and not merely intellectual.

Using a nutritionist introduced a third person into our relationship, toward whom Sophia could feel the negative feelings she denied in relation to me. Initially, Sophia found the nutritionist's advise helpful about food (e.g. creating a food plan), and rules about eating (e.g. more defined eating times; no eating while on the computer or watching TV) and minor modifications of her exercise schedule (e.g. time limits and more variety in her workouts by adding yoga). These changes led to a quick decrease in frequency of her binges, but soon, Sophia's dislike of the nutritionist, although non-verbal, was clear. It was only after I verbalized what I noticed in her tone and gestures, that she let on how critical and rejecting she felt: from how the nutritionist spoke (i.e. insensitive; blunt) to how she dressed (i.e. not very stylish) to how "in shape" she was (i.e. not very). As she spoke, I could hear how she must have experienced her parents' criticism.

Hearing the absolute disdain in her voice, I became concerned that this displaced aggression would lead to non-compliance with the nutritionists' advice. The fact that the transference lacked any strong affect, let alone disdain, led me to ask how she felt about me having referred her to such an incompetent person. She admitted that she had in fact contemplated the same question but explained that when this thought had occurred to her, she had just told herself that I "must not really know the nutritionist". This convenient way of avoiding negative feelings about me was explored in relation to her childhood and current relationships as her way of managing her feelings and others. This also allowed us to explore why she needed to like everything about me and nothing about the nutritionist. These interactions of course required a great deal of verbalization of the therapeutic process on my part, explaining how I understood various situations, as well as inviting her input, consistent with a more active approach (Murphy et al., 2005).

As Sophia's symptoms decreased and she became more aware of her own feelings and reactions to others, she could talk more directly about our relationship. She told me how apprehensive she felt at the thought of talking about feeling angry, hurt or disappointed with me. Simultaneously, she began to have such conversations with her mother and siblings. In treatment, she began to reject some of my interpretations. When I pointed out this new positive development in our relationship she admitted that historically when I had asked whether an interpretation had seemed right to her, she had felt that she must accept it or else face rejection. She explained, "I figured if you said it, it must be right". Her progress was further obvious when she announced one day that she was no longer "superstitious", and explained that the thought of having made progress no longer made her worry that it would all disappear. This seemed to reflect her foot being more firmly planted in reality, with her fears and fantasies having a lesser hold on her. Having a greater sense of efficacy along with lessened need for symptoms were indications for improvement after 12 months of treatment.

4. Conclusions

Treatment of bulimia is often complicated by difficulties in the patient's ability to access emotional experiences, resistance to changing overt symptoms and interpersonal issues enacted with the therapist. Among adolescents, this is further complicated by their limited capacity for expressing abstract concepts such as self-awareness (Golden et al., 2003). Investigation of an integrated psychodynamic approach, where psychodynamic principles and practice are used in tandem with behavioral strategies have yielded positive results (Murphy et al., 2005). Such an approach aims to address symptoms with attention to their role in regulation of the patient's affect and self-esteem, self-efficacy and issues related to separation/individuation with a special attention to the immediate relationship with the therapist. Transference and countertransference are important to consider since the bulimic adolescent has spent her life avoiding being known, while also longing to be known, manifested therapeutically as attempts to control the therapist and preventing an emotional connection. Slow acknowledgement of the enactments within the therapeutic dyad are essential to the success of the integrated treatment, which requires implementation of cognitive and behavioral strategies.

Highlights

- Bulimia results from gender-specific conflicts expressed through the body, i.e., the body takes on a central role for the continuity of the sense of self and is used to express conflicts around dependence and sexuality.
- While Cognitive Behavioral theory considers all ED patients as failing to connect their own behaviors to day-to-day events and negative moods; the psychodynamic perspective expands this idea to include how they fail to understand their behaviors and negative mood in relation to mental states, such as thoughts or feelings – referred to as mentalization, which correlates with attachment.
- An integrated psychodynamic treatment of bulimia expands the CBT-derived hypotheses about cognitions that maintain bulimia to include patients' unconscious operations used to deny unwanted internal states, to regulate affect and to protect the self against fragmentation.
- An integrated psychodynamic approach addresses not only symptoms, but also motivation, insight and resistance while it emphasizes the importance of understanding the emotional reactions of both the patient and the therapist.
- In treatment, attention to therapeutic relationship is central, whereby the therapist uses words to demonstrate authenticity, flexibility, creativity and willingness to take interpersonal risks – in short be the antithesis of the ED patient.

References

Abbate Daga, G., Quaranta, M., Notaro, G., Urani, C., Amianto, F., & Fassino, S. (2011), Terapia familiare e disturbi del comportamento alimentare nelle giovani pazienti: stato dell'arte. *Giornale Italiano di Psicopatologia*, 17, pp. 40–47.

Agras, W.S., & Mascola, A.J. (2005), Risk factors for childhood overweight. *Current Opinion in Pediatrics*, 17 (5), pp. 648–652.

Al-Sendi, A.M., Shetty, P., & Musaiger, A.O. (2003), Prevalence of overweight and obesity among Bahraini adolescents: a comparison between three different sets of criteria. *European Journal of Clinical Nutrition*, 57 (3), pp. 471–474.

Albers, S. (2011), Using mindful eating to treat food restriction: a case study. *Eating Disorders*, 19, pp. 97–107.

Algini, M.L. (Ed.) (2007), *Sulla storia della psicoanalisi infantile in Italia*. Rome, Borla.

Allen, N.B., Chambers, R., & Knight, W. (2006), Mindfulness-based psychotherapies: a review of conceptual foundations, empirical evidence and practical considerations. *The Australian and New Zealand Journal of Psychiatry*, 40 (4), pp. 285–294.

American Psychiatric Association (2013), *Diagnostic and statistical manual of mental disorders, DSM-5*, V ed. Washington DC, American Psychiatric Press; Italian trans., *Manuale diagnostico e statistico dei disturbi mentali, DSM-5*, V ed., Milan, Cortina, 2014.

Ammaniti, M., Lucarelli, L., Cimino, S., D'Olimpio, F., & Chatoor, I. (2010), Maternal psychopathology and child risk factors in infantile anorexia. *International Journal of Eating Disorders*, 43, pp. 233–240.

Ammaniti, M., Lucarelli, L., Cimino, S., D'Olimpio, F., & Chatoor, I. (2012), Feeding disorders of infancy: a longitudinal study to middle childhood. *International Journal of Eating Disorders*, 45, pp. 272–280.

Anderson, C.M., & McMillan, K. (2001), Parental use of escape extinction and differential reinforcement to treat food selectivity. *Journal of Applied Behavior Analysis*, 34 (4), pp. 511–515.

Andolfi, M. (Ed.) (2002), *I pionieri della terapia familiare*. Milan, Franco Angeli.

Aranson, J.K. (1993), *Insights in the psychodynamic psychotherapy of anorexia and bulimia*. Northvale, NJ, Jason Aranson.

Arenz, S., Rückerl, R., Koletzko, B., & von Kries, R. (2004), Breast-feeding and childhood obesity: a systematic review. *International Journal of Obesity*, 28 (10), pp. 1247–1256.

Arfelli Galli, A. (1995), L'istituzione scolastica come laboratorio sociale. *Pedagogia e Vita*, 53, pp. 49–60.

Arfelli Galli, A. (2006), Field–theory and analysis of child behavior in Metzger's school, development to self consciousness and motivation for achievement. *Gestalt Theory*, 28 (4), pp. 389–402.

Asen, E., & Fonagy P. (2012), Mentalization-based therapeutic interventions for families. *Journal of Family Therapy*, 34, pp. 347–370.

Atzaba-Poria, N., Meiri, G., Millikovsky, M., Barkai, A., Dunaevsky-Idan, M., & Yerushalmi, B. (2010), Father–child and mother–child interaction in families with a child feeding disorder: the role of paternal involvement. *Infant Mental Health Journal*, 31, pp. 682–698.

Baer, R.A. (2003), Mindfulness training as a clinical intervention: a conceptual and empirical review. *Clinical Psychology: Science and Practice*, 10 (2), pp. 125–143.

Baker, J.L., Michaelsen, K.F., Rasmussen, K.M., & Sørensen, T.I. (2004), Maternal prepregnant body mass index, duration of breastfeeding, and timing of complementary food introduction are associated with infant weight gain. *The American Journal of Clinical Nutrition*, 80 (6), pp. 1579–1588.

Baker, J.L., Michaelsen, K.F., Sørensen, T.I., & Rasmussen, K.M. (2007), High prepregnant body mass index is associated with early termination of full and any breastfeeding in Danish women. *The American Journal of Clinical Nutrition*, 86 (2), pp. 404–411.

Bakermans-Kranenburg, M.J., Van Ijzendoorn, M.H., & Juffer, F. (2003), Less is more: meta-analyses of sensitivity and attachment interventions in early childhood. *Psychological Bulletin*, 129 (2), pp. 195–215.

Baldaro, B. (2002), Enuresi ed encopresi: segnali di crisi sulla strada dell'autonomia. *Il dolore mentale nel percorso evolutivo*, edited by E. Trombini, Urbino, Quattro Venti.

Baldaro, B., Trombini, E., & Trombini, G. (1994), I sintomi psicosomatici dell'evacuazione come segnali di crisi psicologica nell'infanzia. *Introduzione alla clinica psicologica*, edited by G. Trombini. Bologna, Zanichelli.

Baldaro, B., & Trombini, G. (1989), *Disturbo del controllo degli sfinteri, in Trattato enciclopedico di psicologia dell'età evolutiva*, edited by M.W. Battacchi, Padova, Piccin, vol. 2, tomo 2.

Barker, D.J. (1995). Fetal origins of coronary heart disease. *British Medical Journal*, 311 (6998), pp. 171–174.

Barnett, B. (1995), Preventive intervention: pregnancy and early parenting, in *Handbook of studies in preventive psychiatry*, edited by B. Raphael & G.D. Burows. Amsterdam, Elsevier, pp. 95–120.

Battacchi, M.W., & Giovanelli, G. (1988), *Psicologia dello sviluppo*. Rome, La Nuova Italia Scientifica.

Beebe, B. (2003), Brief mother–infant treatment: psychoanalytically informed video feedback. *Infant Mental Health Journal*, 24 (1), pp. 24–52.

Benoit, D. (1996), Difficoltà di accrescimento e disturbi alimentari, in *Manuale di salute mentale infantile*, edited by C.H. Zeanah. Milan, Masson.

Benoit, D. (2000), Feeding disorders, failure to thrive, and obesity, in *Handbook of infant mental health*, edited by C.H. Zeanah. New York and London, Guilford Press.

Benoit, D., & Coolbear, J. (1998), Post-traumatic feeding disorders in infancy: behaviors predicting treatment outcome. *Infant Mental Health Journal*, 19 (4), pp. 409–421.

Benoit, D., Wang, E.E.L., & Zlotkin, S.H. (2000), Discontinuation of enterostomy tube feeding by behavioral treatment in early childhood: a randomized controlled trial. *The Journal of Pediatrics*, 137 (4), pp. 498–503.

Bion, W. (1962), A theory of thinking. *The International Journal of Psycho-analysis*, 43, pp. 306–310.

Bion, W.R. (1963), Eine Theorie des Denkens. *Psyche – Z Psychoanal*, 17 (7), pp. 426–435.

Blos, P. (1979), The adolescent passage: developmental issues. New York, International Universities Press; Italian trans., *L'adolescenza come fase di transizione. Aspetti e problemi del suo sviluppo*. Rome, Armando, 1988.

Bornstein, R., & Greenberg, G. (1991), Dependency and eating disorders in female psychiatric patients. *Journal of Nervous and Mental Disorders*, 179, pp. 148–152.

Bosello, O., & Cuzzolaro, M. (2013), *Obesità*. Bologna, Il Mulino.

Bosello, O., Donataccio, M.P., & Cuzzolaro, M. (2016), Obesity or obesities? Controversies on the association between body mass index and premature mortality. *Eating and Weight Disorders*, 21, pp. 165–174.

Bosi, R., & Zavattini, G.C. (1982), La preadolescenza nella letteratura psicoanalitica. *Neuropsichiatria infantile*, 256–257, pp. 901–916.

Bowen, M. (1979), *Dalla famiglia all'individuo*; Italian trans., Rome, Astrolabio, 1980.

Brazelton, T.B., & Greenspan, S.I. (2000), The irreducible needs of children, London, Perseus; Italian trans., *I bisogni irrinunciabili dei bambini*. Milan, Cortina, 2001.

Bryant-Waugh, R. (2013), Feeding and eating disorders in children. *Current Opinion in Psychiatry*, 26, pp. 537–542.

Bryant-Waugh, R., Markham, L., Kreipe, R.E., & Walsh, B.T. (2010), Feeding and eating disorders in childhood. *International Journal of Eating Disorders*, 43, pp. 98–111.

Bryant-Waugh, R., & Piepenstock, E.H.C. (2008), Childhood disorders: feeding and related disorders of infancy or early childhood, in *Psychiatry*, edited by A. Tasman, J. Kay, J.A. Lieberman, M.B. First & M. Maj. Chichester, John Wiley & Sons.

Busato Barbaglio, C., & Mondello, M.L. (Eds.) (2011). *Nuovi assetti della clinica picoanalitica in età evolutiva*, Rome, Borla.

Candelori, C., & Trumello, C. (2015), *La consultazione clinica con il bambino*. Bologna, Il Mulino.

Canestrari, R., & Trombini G. (1975), Psychotherapie als Umstrukturierung des Feldes, in *Gestalttheorie in der modernen Psychologie*, edited by S. Ertel, L. Kemmler & M. Stadler. Darmstadt, Steinkopf.

Cardona Cano, S., Tiemeier, H., Van Hoeken, D., Tharner A., Jaddoe, V.W.V., Hofman, A., Verhulst, F.C. & Hoek, H.W. (2015), Trajectories of picky eating during childhood: a general population study. *International Journal of Eating Disorders*, 48 (6), pp. 570–579.

Carr, A. (2014), The evidence base for family therapy and systemic interventions for child-focused problems. *Journal of Family Therapy*, 36, pp. 107–157.

Carson, J.W., Carson, K.M., Gil, K.M., & Baucom, D.H. (2006), Mindfulness-based relationship enhancement (MBRE) in couples, in *Mindfulness-based treatment approaches: clinician's guide to evidence base and applications*, edited by R.A. Baer. Burlington, MA, Elsevier, pp. 309–331.

Casement, P. (1991), *Learning from the patient*. New York, The Guilford Press.

Casper, R.C. (1983), On the emergence of bulimia nervosa as a syndrome: a historical view. *International Journal of Eating Disorders*, 2 (3), pp. 3–16.

Cate, R., Khademi, M., Judd, P., & Miller, H. (2013), Deficits in mentalization as a risk factor for the future development of eating disorders: a pilot study. *Advances in Eating Disorders: Theory, Research and Practice*, 1 (3), pp. 187–194.

Chambers, R., Gullone, E., & Allen, N.B. (2009), Mindful emotion regulation: an integrative review. *Clinical Psychology Review*, 29 (6), pp. 560–572.

Chatoor, I. (1996), Feeding and other disorders of infancy or early childhood, in *Psychiatry*, edited by A. Tasman, J. Kay & L. Lieberman. Philadelphia, PA, Saunders.

Chatoor, I. (2009), *Diagnosis and treatment of feeding disorders in infants, toddlers, and young children*. Washington, DC, Zero-to-Three, National Center for Infants, Toddlers, and Families.

Chatoor, I., Ganiban, J., Harrison, J., & Hirsch, R. (2001), Observation of feeding in the diagnosis of posttraumatic feeding disorder of infancy. *Journal of the American Academy of Child and Adolescent Psychiatry*, 40, pp. 595–602.

Chatoor, I., Ganiban, J., Hirsh, R., Borman-Spurrell, E., & Mrazek, D.A. (2000), Maternal characteristics and toddler temperament in infantile anorexia. *Journal of the American Academy of Child and Adolescent Psychiatry*, 39, pp. 743–751.

Chatoor, I., Ganiban, J., Surles, J., & Doussard-Roosevelt, J. (2004), Physiological regulation and infantile anorexia: a pilot study. *Journal of the American Academy of Child and Adolescent Psychiatry*, 43, pp. 1019–1025.

Cicchetti, D., & Cohen, D.J. (Eds.) (2006), *Developmental psychopathology: theory and method* (2nd ed.). New York, John Wiley & Sons.

Claparède, E. (1930). L'émotion "pure". ["Pure" emotion]. *Archives de Psychologie*, 22, 333–347.

Clawson, E.P., & Elliott, C.A. (2014), Integrating evidence-based treatment of pediatric feeding disorders into clinical practice: challenges to implementation. *Clinical Practice in Pediatric Psychology*, 2 (3), pp. 312–321.

Cohen-Katz, J. (2004), Mindfulness-based stress reduction and family systems medicine: a natural fit. *Families, Systems, and Health*, 22 (2), pp. 204–206.

Cole, T.J., Bellizzi, M.C., Flegal, K.M., & Dietz, W.H., (2000), Establishing a standard definition for child overweight and obesity worldwide: international survey. *British Medical Journal*, 320, pp. 1240–1243.

Cooper, P.J., Whelan, E., Woolgar, M., Morrell, J., & Murray, L. (2004), Association between childhood feeding problems and maternal eating disorder: role of the family environment. *The British Journal of Psychiatry*, 184, pp. 210–215.

Corboz-Warnery, A. (2014), An in-depth look at the LTP and video-feedback, in *The Baby and the couple: Understanding and treating young families*, edited by E. Fivaz-Depeursinge & D.A. Philip. New York, Routledge; Italian trans., *Uno sguardo approfondito al LTP e al video-feedback*, Milan, Cortina, 2015, pp. 169–184.

Costin, C. (2006), *The eating disorders sourcebook: a comprehensive guide to the causes, treatments, and prevention of eating disorders*. New York, Mc Graw-Hill.

Cramer, B. (1998). Mother–infant psychotherapies: a widening scope in technique. *Infant Mental Health Journal*, 19 (2), pp. 151–167.

Cuzzolaro, M. (2014). Eating and weight disorders: Studies on anorexia, bulimia, and obesity turns 19. *Eating and Weight Disorders*, 19, pp. 1–2.

Cuzzolaro, M., Piccolo, F., & Speranza, A.M. (2009), *Anoressia, bulimia, obesità: disturbi dell'alimentazione e del peso corporeo da 0 a 14 anni*. Rome, Carocci.

Dare, C., Eisler, I., Russell, G.F.M., & Szmukler, G.I. (1990), The clinical and theoretical impact of a controlled trial of family therapy in anorexia nervosa. *Journal of Marital and Family Therapy*, 16 (1), pp. 39–57.

Davies, P.T., Cummings, E.M., & Winter, M.A. (2004), Pathways between profiles of family functioning, child security in the interparental subsystem, and child psychological problems. *Development and Psychopathology*, 16, pp. 525–550.

Daws, D. (1997), The perils of intimacy: closeness and distance in feeding and weaning. *Journal of Child Psychotherapy*, 23 (2), pp. 179–199.

de Campora, G., D'Onofrio, E., & Zavattini, G.C. (2014), Fattori di rischio precoci nello sviluppo del sovrappeso in età pediatrica: una rassegna della letteraturai. *Giornale Italiano di Psicologia*, 2, pp. 265–294.

de Campora, G., Giromini, L., Guerriero, V., Chiodo, C., Zavattini, G.C., & Larciprete, G. (2019), Influence of maternal reflective functioning on mothers' and children's weight: A follow-up study. *Infant Mental Health Journal*, 40 (6), pp. 862–873.

de Campora, G., Giromini, L., Larciprete, G., Li Volsi, V., & Zavattini, G.C. (2014), The impact of maternal overweight and emotion regulation on early eating behaviors. *Eating Behaviors*, 15, pp. 403–409.

de Campora, G., Larciprete, G., Delogu, A.M., Meldolesi, C., & Giromini, L. (2016), A longitudinal study on emotion dysregulation and obesity risk: from pregnancy to 3 years of age of the baby. *Appetite*, 96, pp. 95–101.

de Campora, G., & Meldolesi, C. (2014), Indicatori di rischio psicopatologico nel rischio di sovrappeso gestazionale. *Giornale Italiano di Psicologia*, 3, pp. 601–610.

de Campora, G., & Zavattini, G.C. (2011), Il bambino in relazione con il mondo, in *Nuovi assetti della clinica psicoanalitica in età evolutiva*, edited by C. Busato Barbaglio, M.L. Mondello. Rome, Borla.

de Campora, G., & Zavattini, G.C. (2015), Oggetti interni e modelli operativi interni, in *Psicologia dinamica*, edited by G. Amadei, D. Cavanna & G.C. Zavattini. Bologna, Il Mulino.

de Groot, J.M., & Rodin, G. (1994), Eating disorders, female psychology, and the self. *Journal of American Academy of Psychoanalysis*, 22, pp. 299–317.

DiSantis, K.I., Hodges, E.A., Johnson, S.L., & Fisher, J.O. (2011), The role of responsive feeding in overweight during infancy and toddlerhood: a systematic review. *International Journal of Obesity*, 35 (4), pp. 480–492.

Duncan, L.G., Coatsworth, J.D., & Greenberg, M.T. (2009), A model of mindful parenting: implications for parent–child relationships and prevention research. *Clinical Child and Family Psychology Review*, 12, pp. 255–270.

Dunitz-Scheer, M., Marinschek, S., Beckenbach, H., Kratky, E., Hauer, A., & Scheer, P. (2011), Tube-dependency: a reactive eating behavior disorder. *Infant, Child and Adolescent Nutrition*, 3, pp. 209–215.

Eccles, J.S. (1999), The development of children ages 6 to 14. *The Future of Children*, 9 (2), pp. 30–44.

Egeland, B., Weinfeld, N.S., Bosquet, M., & Cheng, V.K. (2000), Remembering, repeating, and working through: lessons from attachment-based interventions, in *WAIMH Handbook of infant mental health*, Vol. 4, edited by J.D. Osofsky & H.E. Fitzgerald. New York, John Wiley & Sons, pp. 38–89.

Eisler, I., Dare, C., Hodes, M., Russell, G., Dodge, E., & Le Grange, D. (2000), Family therapy for adolescent anorexia nervosa: the results of a controlled comparison of two family interventions. *Journal of Child Psychology and Psychiatry*, 41, pp. 727–736.

Eisler, I., le Grange, D., & Asen, E. (2006), Interventi familiari, Italian trans. in *I disturbi dell'alimentazione*, edited by J. Treasure, U. Schmidt & E. van Furth. Bologna, Il Mulino, 2008, pp. 231–258.

Emanuel, L. (2010), Review: *Handbook of infant mental health*, 3rd edition. *Infant Observation*, 13 (2), pp. 249–253.

Erikson, E.H. (1959), *Identity and the life cycle* (Psychological Issues, 1). New York, International Universities Press; Italian trans., *I cicli della vita: continuità e mutamenti*. Rome, Armando, 1991.

Fairburn, C.G. (2008), *Cognitive behavior therapy and eating disorders*. New York, Guilford Press.

Farrell, E. (2001), *Lost for words: the psychoanalysis of anorexia and bulimia*. London, Process Press.

Farrow, C., & Blissett, J. (2006), Does maternal control during feeding moderate early infant weight gain? *Pediatrics*, 118 (2), pp. 293–298.

Farrow, C.V., & Coulthard, H. (2012), Relationships between sensory sensitivity, anxiety and selective eating in children. *Appetite*, 58 (3), pp. 842–846.

Fischer, A.J., Luiselli, J.K., & Dove, M.B. (2015), Effects of clinic and in-home treatment on consumption and feeding-associated anxiety in an adolescent with avoidant/restrictive food intake disorder. *Clinical Practice in Pediatric Psychology*, 3 (2), pp. 154–166.

Fivaz-Depeursinge, E. (2008), Infant's triangular communication in "two for one" versus "two against one" family triangles: case illustrations. *Infant Mental Health Journal*, 29, pp. 189–202.

Fivaz-Depeursinge, E., & Corboz-Warnery, A. (1999), *The primary triangle: a developmental systems view of mothers, fathers, and infants*. New York, Basic Books; trans. It. *Il triangolo primario: le prime interazioni triadiche tra madre, padre e bambino*. Milan, Cortina, 2000.

Fonagy, P., Gergely, G., Jurist, E.L., & Target, M. (2002), *Affect regulation, mentalization, and the development of the self*. New York, Other Press; Italian trans., *Regolazione affettiva, mentalizzazione e sviluppo del Sé*. Milan, Cortina, 2005.

Fonagy, P., & Target, M. (2000), Playing with reality: the persistence of dual psychic reality in borderline patients. *International Journal of Psychoanalysis*, 81, pp. 853–873.

Forney, K.J., Buchman-Schmitt, J.M., Keel, P.K., & Frank, G.K.W. (2016), The medical complications associated with purging. *International Journal of Eating Disorders*, 49 (3), pp. 249–259.

Framson, C., Kristal, A.R., Schenk, J.M., Littman, A.J., Zeliadt, S., & Benitez, D. (2009), Development and validation of the mindful eating questionnaire. *Journal of the American Dietetic Association*, 109 (8), pp. 1439–1444.

Fukkink, R.G. (2008), Video feedback in widescreen: a meta-analysis of family programs. *Clinical Psychology Review*, 28 (6), pp. 904–916.

Galloway, A.T., Fiorito, L., Lee, Y., & Birch, L.L. (2005), Parental pressure, dietary patterns, and weight status among girls who are "picky eaters". *Journal of the American Dietetic Association*, 105, pp. 541–548.

Galloway, A.T., Lee, Y., & Birch, L.L. (2003), Predictors and consequences of food neophobia and pickiness in young girls. *Journal of the American Dietetic Association*, 103, pp. 692–698.

Gambrel, E.L., & Keeling, M.L. (2010), Relational aspects of mindfulness: implications for the practice of marriage and family therapy. *Contemporary Family Therapy*, 32, pp. 412–426.

Germer, C.K. (2005), Teaching mindfulness in psychotherapy, in *Mindfulness and Psychotherapy*, edited by C.K. Germer, R.D. Siegel, P.R. Fulton. New York, Guilford, pp. 113–129.

Gilbert, P. (Ed.). (2005), *Compassion: conceptualisations, research and use in psychotherapy*. London, Routledge.

Golden, N.H., Katzman, D.K., Kreipe, R.E., Stevens, S.L., Sawyer, S.M., Rees, J., & Rome, E.S. (2003), Eating disorders in adolescents: position paper of the Society for Adolescent Medicine. *Journal of Adolescent Health*, 33 (6), pp. 496–503.

Grava, C., Lucarelli L., & Ammaniti, M. (2014), Gli eventi traumatici oroalimentari nell'infanzia: interazioni alimentari madre-bambino e padre-bambino a confronto. *Infanzia e Adolescenza*, 13, pp. 148–160.

Graziano, P.A., Calkins, S.D., & Keane, S.P. (2010), Toddler self-regulation skills predict risk for pediatric obesity. *International Journal of Obesity*, 34 (4), pp. 633–641.

Gueron-Sela, N., Atzaba-Poria, N., Meiri, G., & Yerushalmi, B. (2011), Maternal worries about child underweight mediate and moderate the relationship between child feeding disorders and mother–child feeding interactions. *Journal of Pediatric Psychology*, 36, pp. 827–836.

Hafstad, G.S., Abebe, D.S., Torgersen, L., & von Soest, T. (2013), Picky eating in preschool children: the predictive role of the child's temperament and mother's negative affectivity. *Eating Behaviors*, 14, pp. 274–277.

Haines, J., Kleinman, K.P., Rifas-Shiman, S.L., Field, A.E., & Austin, S.B. (2010). Examination of shared risk and protective factors for overweight and disordered eating among adolescents. *Archives of Pediatric and Adolescent Medicine*, 164 (4), pp. 336–343.

Harder, T., Bergmann, R., Kallischnigg, G., & Plagemann, A. (2005), Duration of breastfeeding and risk of overweight: a meta-analysis. *American Journal of Epidemiology*, 162 (5), pp. 397–403.

Harnett, P.H., & Dawe, S. (2013), The contribution of mindfulness-based therapies for children and families and proposed conceptual integration. *Child and Adolescent Mental Health*, 17 (4), pp. 195–208.

Hartmann, A., Zeeck, A., & Barrett, M.S. (2010), Interpersonal problems in eating disorders. *International Journal of Eating Disorders*, 43, pp. 619–627.

Herkov, M., Greer, R., Blau, B., McGuire, J., & Eaker, D. (1994), Bulimia: an empirical analysis of psychodynamic theory. *Psychological Reports*, 75, pp. 51–56.

Herscovici, C.R., & Bay, L. (1996), Favorable outcome for anorexia nervosa patients treated in Argentina with a family approach. *Eating Disorders: The Journal of Treatment & Prevention*, 4 (1), pp. 59–66.

Hirschmann, J.R., & Zaphiropoulos, L. (2012), *Kids, carrots, and candy: a practical, positive approach to raising children free of food and weight problems*. Scotts Valley, CA, CreateSpace Independent Publishing Platform Publishing.

Institute of Medicine (2009), *Weight gain during pregnancy: reexamining the guidelines*, edited by K.M. Rasmussen & A.L. Yaktine. Committee to Reexamine, IOM.

Jackson, D.D. (1977), Lo studio della famiglia; Italian trans., in *La prospettiva relazionale*, edited by P. Watzlawick & J. Weakland. Rome, Astrolabio, 1978.

Jacobi, C., Schmitz, G., & Stewart, A. (2008), Is picky eating an eating disorder? *International Journal of Eating Disorders*, 41 (7), pp. 626–634.

Jahnke, D.L., & Warschburger, P.A. (2008), Familial transmission of eating behaviors in preschool-aged children. *Obesity*, 16 (8), pp. 1821–1825.

Juffer, F., Bakermans-Kranenburg, M.J., & Van IJzendoorn, M.H. (2008), *Introduction and outline of the VIPP and VIPP-R program. Promoting positive parenting: an attachment-based intervention.* Mahwah, NJ, Erlbaum.

Juffer, F., & Steele, M. (2014), What words cannot say: the telling story of video in attachment-based interventions. *Attachment & Human Development*, 16 (4), pp. 307–314.

Kabat-Zinn, J. (1990), *Full catastrophe living: using the wisdom of your body and mind to face stress, pain and illness.* New York, Delacorte.

Kabat-Zinn, J. (1994), *Wherever you go, there you are: mindfulness mediation in everyday life.* New York, Hyperion.

Kaye, K. (1982), *La vita mentale e sociale del bambino*, Italian trans. Rome, Il Pensiero Scientifico Editore, 1989.

Kaye, W. H., Bulik, C. M., Thornton, L., Barbarich, N., & Masters, K. (2004). Comorbidity of anxiety disorders with anorexia and bulimia nervosa. *American Journal of Psychiatry*, 161, 2215–2221.

Kerns, K.A. (2008), L'attaccamento nella seconda infanzia; Italian trans., in *Manuale dell'attaccamento. Teoria, ricerca e applicazioni cliniche*, edited by J. Cassidy and P. R. Shaver. Rome, Giovanni Fioriti Editore, 2010, pp. 418–436.

Killen, J., Taylor, C., Hayward, C., Wilson, D., Haydel, K., Hammer, L.D., Simmonds, B., Robinson, T.N., Litt, I., Varady, A., & Kraemer, H. (1994), Pursuit of thinness and onset of eating disorder symptoms in a community sample of adolescent girls: a 3 year prospective analysis. *International Journal of Eating Disorders*, 6, pp. 227–238.

King, P. (1978), Affective response of the analyst to the patient's communication. *International Journal of Psychoanalysis*, 59, pp. 9–34.

Klamma, M. (1957), *Über das Selbermachenwollen und Ablehnen von Hilfen bei Kleinkindern*, Unpublished Bachelor thesis, Psychologisches Institut der Universitat Munster, 1957.

Klein, M. (1929), La personificazione nel gioco infantile, in *Scritti (1921–1958)*. Turin, Boringhieri, 1978.

Koren-Karie, N., Oppenheim, D., & Goldsmith, D. (2010), Keeping the inner world of the child in mind, in *Attachment theory in clinical work with children: bridging the gap between research and practice*, edited by D. Oppenheim & D.F. Goldsmith. New York, The Guilford Press; Italian trans., *Tenere nella mente il mondo interno del bambino*. Rome, Borla Edizioni, 2010, pp. 69–97.

Krebs, N.F., Himes, J.H., Jacobson, D., Nicklas, T.A., Guilday, P., & Styne, D. (2007), Assessment of child and adolescent overweight and obesity. *Pediatrics*, 120 (Supplement 4), pp. S193–S228.

Kreisler, L., Fain, M., & Soulè, M. (1974), *L'enfant et son corps*, Paris, PUF.

Kristeller, J.L., Baer, R.A., & Wolever, R. (2006), Mindfulness-based approaches to eating disorders, in *Mindfulness-based treatment approaches*, edited by R.A. Baer. Burlington, MA, Academic Press, pp. 75–91.

Kristeller, J.L., & Hallett, C.B. (1999), An exploratory study of a meditation based intervention for binge eating disorder. *Journal of Health Psychology*, 4, pp. 357–363.

Kristeller, J.L., & Wolever, R.Q. (2011), Mindfulness-based eating awareness treatment (MB-EAT), conceptual basis. *Eating Disorders: The Journal of Treatment & Prevention*, 19, pp. 49–61.

Kuczmarski, R.J., Ogden, C.L., Grummer-Strawn, L.M., Flegal, K.M., Guo, S.S., Wei, R., Mei, Z., Curtin, L.R., Roche, A.F., & Johnson, C.L. (2000), CDC growth charts: United States. *Advance Data*, June 8, 314, pp. 1–27.

Lam, J. (2015), Picky eating in children. *Frontiers in Pediatrics*, 3, 41.

Lang, M., & Rivolta, L. (2015), *Funzione organizzatrice: dall'Io al Sé, in Psicologia dinamica*, edited by G. Amadei, D. Cavanna & G.C. Zavattini. Bologna, Il Mulino.

Lanyado, M., & Horne, A. (2003), *Manuale di psicoterapia dell'infanzia e dell'adolescenza. Approcci psicoanalitici*. Milan, Franco Angeli.

Lask, B., & Bryant-Waugh, R. (2013), *Eating disorders in childhood and adolescence* (4th ed.). London, Routledge.

le Grange, D., & Eisler, I. (2009), Family interventions in adolescent anorexia nervosa. *Child and Adolescent Psychiatric Clinics of North America*, 18, (1), pp. 159–173.

le Grange, D., Eisler, I., Dare, C., & Russell, G. (1992), Evaluation of family treatments in adolescent anorexia nervosa: a pilot study. *International Journal of Eating Disorders*, 12 (4), pp. 347–357.

le Grange, D., & Schmidt, U. (2005), The treatment of adolescents with bulimia nervosa. *Journal of Mental Health*, 14 (6), pp. 587–597.

Lebovici, S., Diatkine, R., & Soulé M., (Eds.) (1990), *Trattato di psichiatria dell'infanzia e dell'adolescenza*. Rome, Borla.

Lebow, J., Sim, L.A., & Kransdorf, L.N. (2015), Prevalence of a history of overweight and obesity in adolescents with restrictive eating disorders. *Journal of Adolescent Health*, 56 (1), pp. 19–24.

Leckman, J.F., & Pine D.S. (2012), Editorial commentary: challenges and potential of DSM-5 and ICD-11 revisions. *Journal of Child Psychology and Psychiatry*, 53, pp. 449–453.

Li, R., Fein, S.B., & Grummer-Strawn, L.M. (2010), Do infants fed from bottles lack self-regulation of milk intake compared with directly breastfed infants? *Pediatrics*, 1 (6), pp. 1386–1393.

Li, R., Jewell, S., & Grummer-Strawn, L. (2003), Maternal obesity and breast-feeding practices. *American Journal of Clinical Nutrition*, 77, pp. 931–936.

Lichtenberg, J.D. (1995), *Psicoanalisi e sistemi motivazionali*. Milan, Raffaello Cortina Editore.

Lieberman, A.F. (2004), Child–parent psychotherapy: a relationship-based approach to the treatment of mental health disorders in infancy and early childhood, in *Treating Parent–Infant Relationship Problems*, edited by A.J. Sameroff, S.C. McDonough & K.L. Rosenblum. New York, Guilford Press, pp. 97–122.

Linehan, M.M. (1987), Dialectical behavior therapy for borderline personality disorder. Theory and method. *Bulletin of the Menninger Clinic*, 51 (3), pp. 261–276.

Linehan, M.M. (1993), *Cognitive-behavioral treatment of borderline personality disorder*. New York, Guilford Press.

Linscheid, T.R. (2006), Behavioral treatments for pediatric feeding disorders. *Behavior Modification*, 30 (1), pp. 6–23.

Lock, J., & le Grange, D. (2001), Can family-based treatment of anorexia nervosa be manualized? *Journal of Psychotherapy Practice and Research*, 10, pp. 253–261.

Lock, J., & le Grange, D. (2013), *Treatment manual for anorexia nervosa: a family based approach* (2nd ed.). New York, Guilford.

Lucarelli, L. (2001), Disturbi dell'alimentazione, in *Manuale di psicopatologia dell'infanzia*, edited by M. Ammaniti. Milan, Cortina.

Lucarelli, L., Cimino, S., D'Olimpio, F., & Ammaniti, M. (2013), Feeding disorders of early childhood: an empirical study of diagnostic subtypes. *International Journal of Eating Disorders*, 46, pp. 147–155.

Lucarelli, L., Simonelli, A., & Ammaniti, M. (2012), Infantile anorexia: dyadic and triadic interactions during feeding and play. *Infant Mental Health Journal*, 3 (Supplement 33), p. 6.

Lukens, C.T., & Silverman, A.H. (2014), Systematic review of psychological interventions for pediatric feeding problems. *Journal of Pediatric Psychology*, 39 (8), pp. 903–917.

Malagoli Togliatti, M., & Cotugno, A. (1996). *Psicodinamica delle relazioni familiari*. Bologna, Il Mulino.

Manikam, R., & Perman, J.A. (2000), Pediatric feeding disorders. *Journal of Clinical Gastroenterology*, 30 (1), pp. 34–46.

Martin, F.E. (1985), The treatment and outcome of anorexia nervosa in adolescents: a prospective study and five year follow up. *Journal of Psychiatric Research*, 19, pp. 509–514.

Marty, P., de M'Uzan, M., & David, C. (1963), *L'investigation psychosomatique*. Paris, Presses Universitaires de France.

Mascola, A.J., Bryson, S.W., & Agras, W.S. (2010), Picky eating during childhood: a longitudinal study to age 11-Years. *Eating Behaviour*, 11 (4), pp. 253–257.

Mayer, R.D. (1994), *Family therapy in the treatment of eating disorders in general practice*. Dissertation. London, Birkbeck College, University of London.

McCartney, E.J., Anderson, C.M., English, C.L., & Horner, R.H. (2005), Effect of brief clinic-based training on the ability of caregivers to implement escape extinction. *Journal of Positive Behavior Interventions*, 7 (1), pp. 18–32.

McDonough, S.C. (2005), Interaction Guidance: An approach for difficult-to-engage families, in *Handbook of Infant Mental Health* (2nd ed.), edited by C.H. Zeanah. New York, Guilford Press, pp. 485–493.

Mehta, U.J., Siega-Riz, A.M., Herring, A.H., Adair, L.S., & Bentley, M.E. (2011), Maternal obesity, psychological factors, and breastfeeding initiation. *Breastfeeding Medicine*, 6 (6), pp. 369–376.

Meins, E., Fernyhough, C., Wainwright, R., Das Gupta, M., Fradley, E., & Tuckey, M. (2002), Maternal mind-mindedness and attachment security as predictors of theory of mind understanding. *Child Development*, 73, pp. 1715–1726.

Menzel, J.E., Schaefer, L.M., Burke, N.L., Mayhew, L.L., Brannick, M.T., & Thompson, J.K. (2010), Appearance-related teasing, body dissatisfaction, and disordered eating: a meta-analysis. *Body Image*, 7, pp. 261–270.

Metzger, W. (2000), *Psicologia per l'educazione*. Rome, Armando.

Mikulincer, M., & Shaver, P.R. (2008), L'attaccamento adulto e la regolazione delle emozioni, Italian trans., in *Manuale dell'attaccamento. Teoria, ricerca e applicazioni cliniche*, edited by J. Cassidy & P.R. Shaver. Rome, Giovanni Fioriti Editore, 2010, pp. 581–614.

Mikulincer, M., & Shaver, P.R. (2008). Adult attachment and affect regulation, in *Handbook of attachment: Theory, research, and clinical applications*, edited by J. Cassidy & P.R. Shaver (Eds.). New York, Guilford Press, pp. 503–531.

Milnes, S.M., Piazza, C.C., & Carroll, T. (2013), Assessment and treatment of pediatric feeding disorders. *Child Nutrition*, 23, pp. 23–26.

Minuchin, S. (1976), *Famiglie e terapia della famiglia*. Rome, Astrolabio.

Minuchin, S., Reiter, M.D., & Borda, C. (2013), The art of family therapy: Challenging and certainties. New York, Routledge, Italian trans., *L'arte della terapia della famiglia*. Rome, Astrabio, 2014.

Minuchin, S., Rosman, B.L., & Baker, L. (1978), Psychosomatic families: anorexia nervosa in context; Italian trans., *Famiglie psicosomatiche. L'anoressia mentale nel contesto familiare*. Rome, Casa Editrice Astrolabio, 1982.

Mitchell, G.L., Farrow, C., Haycraft, E., & Meyer, C. (2013), Parental influences on children's eating behaviour and characteristics of successful parent-focussed interventions. *Appetite*, 60, pp. 85–94.

Molinari, S., & Lappi, R., (1994), Clinica psicologica e sofferenza psichica. La vita affettiva e le sue radici infantili, in *Introduzione alla clinica psicologica*, edited by G. Trombini. Bologna, Zanichelli.

Moreno, K. (1998), Long-term psychodynamic group psychotherapy for eating disorders: a descriptive case report. *Journal for Specialists in Group Work*, 23 (3), pp. 269–284.

Minuchin, S., Rosman, B.L., & Baker, L., (1980). *Famiglie psicosomatiche*. Rome, Astrolabio.

Murphy, S., Russell, L., & Waller, G. (2005), Integrated psychodynamic psychotherapy for Bulimia Nervosa and Bing Eating Disorder: theory, practice and preliminary findings. *European Eating Disorders Review*, 13, pp. 383–391.

Murray, S.B., Griffiths, S., & le Grange, D. (2014), The role of collegial alliance in family-based treatment of adolescent anorexia nervosa: a pilot study. *International Journal of Eating Disorders*, 47 (4), pp. 418–421.

Must, A., Dallal, G.E., & Dietz, W.H. (1991), Reference data for obesity: 85th and 95th percentiles of body mass index (wt/ht^2) and triceps skinfold thickness. *The American Journal of Clinical Nutrition*, 53, pp. 839–846.

Najdowski, A.C., Wallace, M.D., Doney, J.K., & Ghezzi, P.M. (2003), Parental assessment and treatment of food selectivity in natural settings. *Journal of Applied Behavior Analysis*, 36 (3), pp. 383–386.

Najdowski, A.C., Wallace, M.D., Reagon, K., Penrod, B., Higbee, T.S., & Tarbox, J. (2010), Utilizing a home-based parent training approach in the treatment of food selectivity. *Behavioral Interventions*, 25 (2), pp. 89–107.

National Institute for Health and Care Excellence (NICE) (2004), *Eating disorders: core interventions in the treatment and management of anorexia nervosa, bulimia nervosa and related disorders*, Clinical Guideline, no. 9. London, National Collaborating Centre for Medical Health.

NCD Risk Factor Collaboration (NCD-RisC) (2016), Trends in adult body-mass index in 200 countries from 1975 to 2014: a pooled analysis of 1698 population-based measurement studies with 19·2 million participants. *Lancet*, 387 (10026), pp. 1377–1396.

Neri, N., & Latmiral, S. (Eds.) (2004), *Uno spazio per i genitori*. Rome, Borla.

Nicholls, D., & Bryant-Waugh, R. (2009), Eating disorders of infancy and childhood: Definition, symptomatology, epidemiology, and comorbidity, *Child and Adolescent Psychiatric Clinics of North America*, 18 (1), pp. 17–30.

Nicholls, D., & Jaffa, T. (2007), *Selective eating and other atypical eating problems, in Eating Disorders in Children*, edited by T. Jaffa and B. McDermott. Cambridge, Cambridge University Press, pp. 144–157.

Nielsen, S., & Bará-Carrill, N. (2006), Famiglia, peso della cura e conseguenze sociali; Italian trans., in *I disturbi dell'alimentazione*, edited by J. Treasure, U. Schmidt, & E. van Furth. Bologna, Il Mulino, 2008, pp. 231–258.

Oddy, W.H., Li, J., Landsborough, L., Kendall, G.E., Henderson, S. & Downie, J. (2006), The association of maternal overweight and obesity with breastfeeding duration. *Journal of Pediatrics*, 149, pp. 185–191.

Ogden, C.L., Carroll, M.D., & Flegal, K.M. (2003), Epidemiologic trends in overweight and obesity. *Endocrinology and Metabolism Clinics*, 32 (4), pp. 741–760.

Okada, A., Tsukamoto, C., Hosogi, M., Yamanaka, E., Watanabe, K., Ootyou, K., & Morishima, T. (2007), A study of psychopathology and treatment of children with phagophobia. *Acta Medica Okayama*, 61, pp. 261–269.

Olds, D.L., Eckenrode, J., Henderson, C.R., Kitzman, H., Powers, J., Cole, R., Sidora, L., Morris, P., Pettitt, L.M., & Luckey, D. (1997), Long-term effects of home visitation on maternal life course and child abuse and neglect: fifteen-year follow-up of a randomized trial. *JAMA*, 278 (8), pp. 637–643.

Olds, D.L., & Kitzman, H. (1990), Can home visitation improve the health of women and children at environmental risk? *Pediatrics*, 86 (1), pp. 108–116.

Onnis, L. (2004), *Il Tempo Sospeso. Anoressia e bulimia tra individuo, famiglia e società*. Milan, Franco Angeli.

Owen, C.G., Martin, R.M., Whincup, P.H., Smith, G.D., & Cook, D.G. (2005), Effect of infant feeding on the risk of obesity across the life course: a quantitative review of published evidence. *Pediatrics*, 115, pp. 1367–1377.

Papoušek, M. (2007), Communication in early infancy: an arena of intersubjective learning. *Infant Behaviour and Development*, 30, pp. 258–266.

Patton, C. (1992), Fear of abandonment and binge eating: a subliminal psychodynamic activation investigation. *Journal of Nervous and Mental Disease*, 180, pp. 484–490.

Patton, G.C., Selzer, R., Coffey, C.C.J.B., Carlin, J.B., & Wolfe, R. (1999), Onset of adolescent eating disorders: population based cohort study over 3 years. *British Medical Journal*, 318 (7186), pp. 765–768.

Pepping, C.A., O'Donovan, A., Zimmer-Gembeck, M.J., & Hanisch, M. (2014), Is emotion regulation the process underlying the relationship between low mindfulness and psychosocial distress? *Australian Journal of Psychology*, 66 (2), pp. 130–138.

Perepletchikova, F., & Goodman, G. (2014), Two approaches to treating preadolescent children with severe emotional and behavioral problems: dialectical behavior therapy adapted for children and mentalization-based child therapy. *Journal of Psychotherapy Integration*, 24 (4), pp. 298–312.

Perkins, S., Schmidt, U., Eisler, I., Treasure, J., Yi, I., Winn, S., Robinson, P., Murphy, R., Keville, S., Johnson-Sabine, E., Jenkins, M., Frost, S., Dodge, L., & Berelowitz, M. (2005), Why do adolescents with bulimia nervosa choose not to involve their parents in treatment? *European Child & Adolescent Psychiatry*, 14 (7), pp. 376–385.

Pizzo, B., Williams, K.E., Paul, C., & Riegel, K. (2009), Jump start exit criterion: exploring a new model of service delivery for the treatment of childhood feeding problems. *Behavioral Interventions*, 24 (3), pp. 195–203.

Puliafico, A.C., Comer, J.S., & Albano, A.M. (2013), Coaching approach behavior and leading by modeling: rationale, principles, and a session-by-session description of the CALM Program for early childhood anxiety. *Cognitive and Behavioral Practice*, 20 (4), pp. 517–528.

Quagliata, E., (2002), *Un bisogno vitale. L'importanza del rapporto alimentare nello sviluppo del bambino*. Rome, Casa Editrice Astrolabio.

Reilly, J.J. (2002), Assessment of childhood obesity: national reference data or international approach? *Obesity Research*, 10 (8), pp. 838–840.

Ringer, F., & Crittenden, P.M. (2007), Eating disorders and attachment: the effects of hidden family processes on eating disorders. *European Eating Disorders Review*, 15 (2), pp. 119–130.

Riva Crugnola, C. (2007), *Il bambino e le sue relazioni. Attaccamento e individualità tra teoria e osservazione*. Milan, Cortina.

Robin, A.L., Siegel, P.T., Moye, A.W., Gilroy, M., Dennis, A.B., & Sikand, A. (1999), A controlled comparison of family versus individual therapy for adolescents with anorexia nervosa. *Journal of the American Academy of Child and Adolescent Psychiatry*, 38 (12), pp. 1482–1489.

Rosenblum, K.L., Dayton, C., & McDonough, S.C. (2006), Communicating feelings: links between mothers' representations of their infants, parenting, and infant emotional development, in *Parenting representations: theory, research, and clinical implications*, edited by O. Mayseless. New York, Cambridge University Press, pp. 109–148.

Salomon, J.A., Wang, H., Freeman, M.K., Vos, T., Flaxman, A.D., Lopez, A.D., & Murray, C.J. (2012), Healthy life expectancy for 187 countries, 1990–2010: a systematic analysis for the Global Burden Disease Study 2010. *Lancet*, 380 (9859), pp. 2144–2162.

Sameroff, A.J. (2004), Vie di ingresso e dinamiche degli interventi effettuati sulla relazione madre-bambino; Italian trans., in *Il trattamento clinico della relazione genitore bambino*, edited by A.J. Sameroff, S.C. McDonough & K.L. Rosenblum. Bologna, Il Mulino, pp. 23–50.

Sameroff, A.J. (2010), A unified theory of development: a dialectic integration of nature and nurture. *Child Development*, 81, pp. 6–22.

Sameroff, A.J., DcDonough, S.C., & Rosenblum, K.L. (Eds.) (2004). *Il trattamento clinico delle relazioni genitore/bambino*. Bologna, Il Mulino, 2006.

Sander, L.W. (1991), Paradox and resolution: from the beginning, in *Handbook of child and adolescent psychiatry*, edited by J.D. Noshpitz, S. Greenspan, S. Wieder & J. Osofsky. New York, John Wiley & Sons, vol. 1, section II, pp. 153–160.

Sander, L.W. (2007), Italian trans., *Sistemi viventi. L'emergere della persona attraverso l'evoluzione della consapevolezza*. Milan, Cortina.

Satir, D., Thompson-Brenner, H., Boisseau, C., & Crisafullu, A. (2009), Countertransference reactions to adolescents with eating disorders: relationships to clinician and patient factors. *International Journal of Eating Disorders*, 42 (6), pp. 511–521.

Schmidt, U., Lee, S., Beecham, J., Perkins, S., Treasure, J., Yi, I., Winn, S., Robinson, P., Murphy, R., Keville, S., Johnson-Sabine, E., Jenkins, M., Frost, S., Dodge, L., Berelowitz, M., & Eisler, I. (2007), A randomized controlled trial of family therapy and cognitive behavior therapy guided self-care for adolescents with Bulimia Nervosa and related disorders. *American Journal of Psychiatry*, 164, pp. 591–598.

Seiverling, L., Williams, K., Sturmey, P., & Hart, S. (2012), Effects of behavioral skills training on parental treatment of children's food selectivity. *Journal of Applied Behavior Analysis*, 45 (1), pp. 197–203.

Selvini Palazzoli, M., Boscolo, L., Cecchin, G., & Prata, G. (1980), Ipotizzazione, circolarità, neutralità. *Terapia Familiare*, 7, pp. 7–19.

Selvini Palazzoli, M., Cirillo, S., Selvini, M., & Sorrentino, A.M. (1988), *I giochi psicotici nella famiglia*. Milan, Raffaello Cortina Editore.

Selvini Palazzoli, M., Cirillo, S., Selvini, M., & Sorrentino, A.M. (1998), *Ragazze anoressiche e bulimiche. La terapia familiare*. Milan, Raffaello Cortina Editore.

Senra, C., Sanchez-Cao, E., Seoane, G., & Leung, F. (2006), Evolution of self-concept deficits in patients with eating disorders: the role of family concern about weight and appearance. *European Eating Disorders Review*, 15 (2), pp. 131–138.

Shank, L.M., Tanofsky-Kraff, M., Nelson, E.E., Shomaker, L.B., Ranzenhofer, L.M., Hannallah, L.M., Field, S.E., Vannucci, A., Bongiorno, D.M., Brady, S.M., Condarco, T., Demidowich, A., Kelly, N.R., Cassidy, O., Simmons, W.K., Engel, S.G., Pine, D.S., & Yanovski, J.A. (2015), Attentional bias to food cues in youth with loss of control eating. *Appetite*, 87, pp. 68–75.

Sharp, W.G., Burrell, T.L., & Jaquess, D.L. (2014), The Autism MEAL Plan: a parent-training curriculum to manage eating aversions and low intake among children with autism. *Autism*, 18 (6), pp. 712–722.

Siegel, D.J. (2007), *The mindful brain*. New York, W.W. Norton.

Sifneos, P.E. (1973), The prevalence of 'alexithymic' characteristics in psychosomatic patients. *Psychotherapy and Psychosomatics*, 22, pp. 255–262.

Skarderud, F. (2007), Eating one's words, part I: 'Concretized metaphors' and reflective function in anorexia nervosa – an interview study. *European Eating Disorders Review*, 15, pp. 163–174.

Slade, A. (2010), *Relazione genitoriale e funzione riflessiva. Teoria, clinica e intervento sociale*; Italian trans. Rome, Astrolabio.

Sleddens, E.F., Kremers, S.P., De Vries, N.K., & Thijs, C. (2010), Relationship between parental feeding styles and eating behaviours of Dutch children aged 6–7. *Appetite*, 54 (1), pp. 30–36.

Smith, K., Hill, S., & Bambra, C. (2016), *Health inequalities: Critical perspectives*. Oxford, Oxford University Press.

Solter, A. (2007), A case study of traumatic stress disorder in a 5-month-old infant following surgery. *Infant Mental Health Journal*, 28 (1), pp. 76–96.

Sroufe, L.A. (1990), An organization perspective on the self, in *The self in transition: infancy to childhood*, edited by D. Cicchetti & M. Beeghly. Chicago, IL, University of Chicago Press, pp. 281–307.

Stark, L.J., Powers, S.W., Jelalian, E., Rape, R.N., & Miller, D.L. (1994), Modifying problematic mealtime interactions of children with cystic fibrosis and their parents via behavioral parent training. *Journal of Pediatric Psychology*, 19 (6), pp. 751–768.

Stein, A., Woolley, H., & McPherson, K. (1999), Conflict between mothers with eating disorders and their infants during mealtimes. *The British Journal of Psychiatry*, 175, pp. 455–461.

Stein, A., Woolley, H., Senior, R., Hertzmann, L., Lovel, M., Lee, J., Cooper, S., Wheatcroft, R., Challacombe, F., Patel, P., Nicol-Harper, R., Menzes, P., Schmidt, A., Juszczak, E., & Fairburn, C.G. (2006), Treating disturbances in the relationship between mothers with bulimic eating disorders and their infants: a randomized, controlled trial of video feedback. *American Journal of Psychiatry*, 163 (5), pp. 899–906.

Steinhausen, H.C. (2009), Outcome of eating disorders, *Child and Adolescent Psychiatric Clinics of North America*, 18 (1), pp. 225–242.

Stern, D.N. (1985), *The motherhood constellation: a unified view of parent–infant psychotherapy*. New York, Basic Books.

Stern, D.N. (1989), La rappresentazione dei modelli di relazione: considerazioni evolutive, in *Relationships disturbances in early childhood: a devolpmental approch*, edited by A.J. Sameroff & R.N. Emde. New York, Basic Books; Italian trans., *I disturbi delle relazioni nella prima infanzia*, Turin, Bollati Boringhieri, 1991.

Stern, D.N. (1992), *Il mondo interpersonale del bambino*. Turin, Bollati Boringhieri.

Stern, D.N. (1995), Self/Other differentiation in the domain of intimate socio-affective interaction: some considerations, in *The self in infancy: theory and research*, edited by P. Rochat. Amsterdam, Elsevier, pp. 419–429.

Stern, D.N. (2004), The motherhood constellation: therapeutic approaches to early relational problems, in *Treating parent–infant relationship problems: strategies for intervention*, edited by A.J. Sameroff, S.C. McDonough & K.L. Rosenblum. New York, Guilford Press, pp. 29–43.

Stern, D.N. (2005), *Il momento presente*. Milan, Raffaello Cortina Editore.

Stern, D.N. (2010), *Forms of vitality: exploring dynamic experience in psychology, the arts, psychotherapy, and development*. Oxford, Oxford University Press; Italian trans., *Le forme vitali. L'esperienza dinamica in psicologia, nell'arte, in psicoterapia e nello sviluppo*. Milan, Cortina, 2011.

Strober, M., Lampert, C., Morell, W., Burroughs, J., & Jacobs, C. (1990), A controlled family study of anorexia nervosa: evidence of familial aggregation and lack of shared transmission with affective disorders. *International Journal of Eating Disorders*, 9, pp. 239–253.

Sugarman, A., & Kurash, C. (1982), The body as a transitional object in bulimia. *International Journal of Eating Disorders*, 1 (4), pp. 57–67.

Swanson, S.A., Crow, S.J., le Grange, D., Swendsen, J., & Merikangas, K.R. (2011), Prevalence and correlates of eating disorders in adolescents: results from the national comorbidity survey replication adolescent supplement. *Archives of General Psychiatry*, 68 (7), pp. 714–723.

Tacón, A.M., Caldera, Y.M., & Ronaghan, C. (2004), Mindfulness-based stress reduction in women with breast cancer. *Families, Systems & Health*, 22, pp. 193–203.

Tan, C.C., & Holub, S.C. (2011), Children's self-regulation in eating: associations with inhibitory control and parents' feeding behavior. *Journal of Pediatric Psychology*, 36 (3), pp. 340–345.

Tanofsky-Kraff, M., Marcus, M.D., Yanovski, S.Z., & Yanovski, J.A. (2008), Loss of control eating disorder in children age 12 years and younger: proposed research criteria. *Eating Behaviors*, 9 (3), pp. 360–365.

Tanofsky-Kraff, M., Shomaker, L.B., Wilfley, D.E., Young, J.F., Sbrocco, T., Stephens, M., Ranzenhofer, L.M., Elliott, C., Brady, S., Radin, R.M., Vannucci, A., Bryant, E.J., Osborn, R., Berger, S.S., Olsen, C., Kozlosky, M., Reynolds, J.C., & Yanovski, J.A. (2014), Targeted prevention of excess weight gain and eating disorders in high-risk adolescent girls: a randomized controlled trial. *The American Journal of Clinical Nutrition*, 100 (4), pp. 1010–1018.

Tarbox, J., Schiff, A., & Najdowski, A.C. (2010), Parent-implemented procedural modification of escape extinction in the treatment of food selectivity in a young child with autism. *Education and Treatment of Children*, 33 (2), pp. 223–234.

Task Force on Research Diagnostic Criteria: Infancy and Preschool (2003), Research diagnostic criteria for infants and preschool children: the process and empirical support. *Journal of the American Academy of Child and Adolescent Psychiatry*, 42, pp. 1504–1512.

Taveras, E.M., Rifas-Shiman, S.L., Scanlon, K.S., Grummer-Strawn, L.M., Sherry, B., & Gillman, M.W. (2006), To what extent is the protective effect of breastfeeding on future overweight explained by decreased maternal feeding restriction? *Pediatrics*, 118 (6), pp. 2341–2348.

Taylor, C.M., Wernimont, S.M., Northstone, K., & Emmett, P.M. (2015), Picky/fussy eating in children: review of definitions, assessment, prevalence and dietary intakes. *Appetite*, 95, pp. 349–359.

Telch, C.F., Agras, W.S., & Linehan, M.M. (2000), Group dialectical behavior therapy for binge-eating disorder: a preliminary, uncontrolled trial. *Behavior Therapy*, 31 (3), pp. 569–582.

Tharner, A., Jansen, P.W., Kiefte-de Jong, J.C., Moll, H.A., van der Ende, J., Jaddo, V. W.V., Hofman, A., Tiemeier, H., & Franco, O.H. (2014), Toward an operative diagnosis of fussy/picky eating: a latent profile approach in a population-based cohort. *International Journal of Behavioral Nutrition and Physical Activity*, 11, p. 14.

Thiels, C., & Deb, K.S. (2014). EDDA: An eating disorder diagnostic algorithm according to ICD-11. *Eating and Weight Disorders*, 19(1), pp. 111–114.

Thompson, J.K., & Stice, E. (2001), Thin–ideal internalization: mounting evidence for a new risk factor for body-image disturbance and eating pathology. *Current Directions in Psychological Science*, 10, pp. 181–183.

Thompson-Brenner, H., Weingeroff, J., & Westen, D. (2009), Empirical support for psychodynamic psychotherapy for eating disorders, in *Handbook of evidence based psychodynamic psychotherapy*, edited by R.A. Levy & J.S. Ablon. New York, Humana Press.

Thompson-Brenner, H., & Westen, D. (2005). A naturalistic study of psychotherapy for bulimia nervosa, part 1: comorbidity and therapeutic outcome. *The Journal of Nervous and Mental Disease*, 193 (9), 573–584.

Trevarthen, C. (1990), Le emozioni intuitive: l'evoluzione del loro ruolo nella comunicazione tra madre e bambino, in *Affetti natura e sviluppo delle relazioni interpersonali*, edited by M. Ammaniti & N. Dazzi. Bari, Editore Laterza.

Trevarthen, C. (1998), The concept and foundations of infant intersubjectivity, in *Intersubjective communication and emotion in early ontogeny*, edited by S. Braten. Cambridge, Cambridge University Press, pp. 15–46.

Trevarthen, C., & Aitken, K.J. (2001), Intrinsic motives for companionship in understanding: their origin, development, and significance for infant mental health. *Infant Mental Health Journal*, 22, pp. 95–131.

Troisi, A., Di Lorenzo, G., Alcini, S., Nanni, R., Di Pasquale, C., & Siracusano, A. (2006), Body dissatisfaction in women with eating disorders: relationship to early separation anxiety and insecure attachment. *Psychosomatic Medicine*, 68, pp. 449–453.

Troisi, A., Massaroni, P., & Cuzzolaro, M. (2005), Early separation anxiety and adult attachment style in women with eating disorders. *British Journal of Clinical Psychology*, 44, pp. 89–97.

Trombini, E. (2002), L'opposizione infantile. Ostinazione e protesta psicosomatica, in *Quaderni di Scienze dell'Interazione*, 2, Padova, Upsel Domeneghini Editore.

Trombini, E. (2008), *Psicoterapia dei disturbi alimentari ed evacuativi in età prescolare.* Macerata, SIMPLE.

Trombini, E. (2010), *Il cibo nella camera d'ascolto. I disturbi alimentari precoci e la Giocoterapia Focale con bambini e genitori.* Bologna, Pendragon.

Trombini, E. (2011), Disturbi alimentari ed evacuativi in età prescolare. *Quaderni Di Psicoterapia Infantile*, 63, pp. 123–139.

Trombini, E., De Pascalis, L., & Neri, E. (2015), La giocoterapia focale in età pre-scolare. Il ruolo dei genitori, in *Paternitas sine suffragio. Infanzia. Il padre nella teoria psicodinamica. Contributi teorici e pratica clinica*, edited by G. Pallaoro, I. Vescogni & M. Carione. Rome, IF Press, pp. 117–132.

Trombini, E., & Trombini, G. (2006). Focal play-therapy in the extended child–parents context: a clinical case. *Gestalt Theory*, 28 (4), pp. 375–388.

Trombini, E., & Trombini, G. (2007), Focal play-therapy and eating behavior self-regulation in preschool children. *Gestalt Theory*, 29 (4), pp. 294–301.

Trombini, G. (1969), Sull'esistenza e comparsa della motivazione a fare-da-solo nel campo alimentare ed evacuatorio. *Rivista di Psicologia*, 2, pp. 111–131.

Trombini, G. (1970), Das Selbermachenwollen des Kindes im Bereich der Ernährung und Entleerung, *Prax. Kinderpsichol.*, 19, pp. 1–10.

Trombini, G. (Ed.) (1994), *Introduzione alla clinica psicologica.* Bologna, Zanichelli.

Tsiantis, J., Boethious, S.B., Hallerfors, B., Horne, A., & Tischler, L. (2002). *Il lavoro con i genitori.* Rome, Borla.

Vallino, D. (1998), *Raccontami una storia.* Rome, Borla.

Vallino, D. (2000), Introduzione, in *La "storia" e il "luogo immaginario"*, edited by A. Ferro & F. Borgogno. Rome, Borla.

Vallino, D. (2002a), Per una cultura del legame mentale tra genitori e figli, in *Il dolore mentale nel percorso evolutivo*, edited by E. Trombini, Urbino, Quattro Venti.

Vallino, D. (2002b), La consultazione partecipata. *Rivista di Psicoanalisi*, 48 (2), pp. 325–343.

Vallino, D. (2004), *Pensieri sul gioco dall'Infant Observation*, VII International Infant Observation Conference, Florence, Convitto della Calza, 15–18 April.

Vallino, D. (2007), L'avvio della consultazione partecipata, in *Sulla storia della psicoanalisi infantile in Italia*, edited by M.L. Algini. Rome, Borla.

Vallino, D. (2009), *Fare psicoanalisi con genitori e bambini.* Rome, Borla.

Vallino, D. (2012), Revisiting some lessons learned from Martha Harris, in *Enabling and Inspiring. A tribute to Martha Harris*, in collaboration with M. Rhode, M. Rustin & G.P. Williams, edited by M.H. Williams. London, Karnac, pp. 153–162.

Vallino, D., & Macciò, M. (2004). *Essere neonati.* Rome, Borla.

Vallino, D., & Macciò, M. (Eds.) (2011), *Famiglie, Quaderni di psicoterapia infantile*, no. 63, Roma, Borla.

Vallino, D., & Macciò, M. (Eds.) (2012), *Infant observation–infant research: storie cliniche, applicazioni, ricerche.* Rome, Borla.

von Kries, R., Toschke, A.M., Koletzko, B., & Slikker, W. (2002), Maternal smoking during pregnancy and childhood obesity. *American Journal of Epidemiology*, 156 (10), pp. 954–961.

Wachs, K., & Cordova, J.V. (2007), Mindful relating: exploring mindfulness and emotion repertoires in intimate relationships. *Journal of Marital and Family Therapy*, 33 (4), pp. 464–481.

Wallin, D.J. (2007). *Attachment in psychotherapy*. New York, Guilford Press.

Wang, Y. (2004), Epidemiology of childhood obesity – methodological aspects and guidelines: what is new? *International Journal of Obesity*, 28, pp. S21–S28.

Ward, A., Ramsay, R., Turnbull, S., Benedettini, M., & Treasure, J. (2000), Attachment patterns in eating disorders: past in the present. *International Journal of Eating Disorders*, 28, pp. 370–376.

Watson, P., Wiers, R.W., Hommel, B., Ridderinkhof, K.R., & de Wit, S. (2016), An associative account of how the obesogenic environment biases adolescents' food choices. *Appetite*, 96, pp. 560–571.

Watzlawick, P., & Beavin, J. (1967), Some formal aspects of communication. *American Behavioral Scientist*, 10 (8), pp. *4–8*.

Weden, M.M., Brownell, P., & Rendall, M.S. (2012), Prenatal, perinatal, early life, and sociodemographic factors underlying racial differences in the likelihood of high body mass index in early childhood. *American Journal of Public Health*, 102 (11), pp. 2057–2067.

Whitaker, R.C. (2011), The childhood obesity epidemic: lessons for preventing socially determined health conditions. *Archives of Pediatrics & Adolescent Medicine*, 165 (11), pp. 973–975.

WHO Multicentre Growth Reference Study Group (2006), WHO Child Growth Standards based on length/height, weight and age. *Acta paediatrica*, S450, pp. 76–85.

Wildes, J.E., Kalarchian, M.A., Marcus, M.D., Levine, M.D., & Courcoulas, A.P. (2008). Childhood maltreatment and psychiatric morbidity in bariatric surgery candidates. *Obesity Surgery*, 18 (3), pp. 306–313.

Wilksch, S.M. (2015), School-based eating disorder prevention: a pilot effectiveness trial of teacher-delivered Media Smart. *Early Intervention in Psychiatry*, 9 (1), pp. 21–28.

William, G. (1997), *Internal landscapes and foreign bodies: eating disorders and other pathologies*. London, Duckworth.

Williams, K.E., Riegel, K., Gibbons, B., & Field, D.G., (2007), Intensive behavioral treatment for severe feeding problems: a cost-effective alternative to tube feeding. *Journal of Developmental and Physiological Disabilities*, 17, pp. 299–309.

Winn, S., Perkins, S., Walwyn, R., Schmidt, U., Eisler, I., Treasure, J., Berelowitz, M., Dodge, L., Frost, S., Jenkins, M., Johnson-Sabine, E., Keville, S., Murphy, R., Robinson, P., & Yi, I. (2007), Predictors of mental health problems and negative caregiving experiences in carers of adolescents with bulimia nervosa. *International Journal of Eating Disorders*, 40 (2), pp. 171–178.

Winnicott, D.W. (1965), *The family and individual development*. London, Tavistock; Italian trans., *La famiglia e lo sviluppo dell'individuo*. Rome, Armando, 1968.

Winnicott, D.W. (1971), *Gioco e realtà*; Italian trans. Rome, Armando Editore, 1974.

Winnicott, D.W. (1988), *Sulla natura umana*. Milan, Raffaello Cortina Editore, 1989.

Wolever, R.Q., & Best, J.L. (2009), Mindfulness-based approaches to eating disorders, in *Clinical handbook of mindfulness*, edited by F. Didonna. New York, Springer, pp. 259–288.

Wright, P., Fawcett, J., & Crow, R. (1980), The development of differences in the feeding behaviour of bottle and breast fed human infants from birth to two months. *Behavioural Processes*, 5 (1), pp. 1–20.

Yarock, S.R. (1993), Understanding chronic bulimia: a four psychologies approach. *The American Journal of Psychoanalysis*, 53 (1), pp. 3–17.

Young, J.E., Klosko, J.S., & Weishaar, M.E. (2003). *Schema therapy: a practitioner's guide*. New York, Guilford Press.

Zerbe, K. (2001), The crucial role of psychodynamic understanding in the treatment of eating disorders. *Psychiatric Clinics of North America*, 24, pp. 305–313.

Zero-to-Three National Center for Infants, Toddlers and Families (2005), *Diagnostic classification of mental health and developmental disorders of infancy and early childhood: Revised edition (DC:0–3R)*, Washington DC, Zero-to-Three; Italian trans., *CD:0–3R 1^A Revisione Classificazione diagnostica della salute mentale e dei disturbi di sviluppo nell'infanzia*. Rome, Fioriti, 2008.

Zucker, M., Spinazzola, J., Blaustein, M., & Van der Kolk, B.A. (2006), Dissociative symptomatology in posttraumatic stress disorder and disorders of extreme stress. *Journal of Trauma & Dissociation*, 7 (1), pp. 19–31.

Index

age when symptoms appear, 13
alexithymia, xvi
anorexia nervosa, 75–76
    parent–child interactions and clinical
        intervention, 43–44
antecedents, 12–14, 17
anxiety, 41, 74
    case material, 48, 49, 93
    intervention for reducing, 14
    PTED and, 42, 47
    separation, 41, 47–49
    See also cases: Sophia
applied behaviour analysis (ABA), 12–14
attachment, 25, 33, 34
attachment security, 72–73, 77, 87, 91
    insecure attachment style, 91, 93–95
attachment theory, 14–15, 18
autonomy, 67
    in food collection and intake, 5
avoidant/restrictive food intake disorder
    (ARFID), 13, 36
    relevant clinical aspects of, 36–43

Barker, D.J., 6–7
Barnett, B., 24
binge eating disorder (BED), 23, 77, 92
bingeing, 90, 91. *See also* cases: Sophia
Bion, Wilfred, xv–xvi, 5. *See also* reverie
biopsychosocial approach, 12
body mass index (BMI), xiii, 21–23
boundaries
    family dynamics and, 75, 83
    pre-adolescence and, 72–73
Bowen, Murray, 88n5
breastfeeding, 23, 24
    case material, 45, 48–49, 81, 82
    obese mothers and, 7, 23
    protective effects, 23–24, 88n3

bulimia and adolescence, 90–91, 96–97
    case discussion, 93–96
    clinical approach, 91–93

cases
    Aldo and puppet Lewie (L)/Therapist
        (T), 56, 60–64
    Cloe and puppet Phil/therapist, 61–62
    Francesca and Ms M., 43–44
    Roberto (Rb) and puppet Lewie
        (L)/Therapist (T), 65–68
    Sandro and Ms & Mr A, 79–85
    Sara and Matteo: a story of "power,"
        26–30
    Sophia, 93–96
    Tiziana, 48–49
circularity and circular dynamics, 8, 76, 87
Claparède, Édouard, xv
cognitive-behavioural theory (CBT), 14,
    88n8, 91, 92
cognitive-behavioural therapy (CBT), 91–93
Cohen-Katz, J., 86
compassion, 78
    components/attributes of, 88n9
curiosity, 76, 87

designated patient and the family system,
    75, 80
developmental paradox, 34
*Diagnostic and Statistical Manual of
    Mental Disorders, Fifth Edition*
    (DSM-5), 36
Diagnostic Classification of Mental
    Health and Developmental Disorders
    of Infancy and Early Childhood-
    Revised (DC: 0–3R), 36, 37t, 40, 50n2
dialectical behaviour therapy (DBT), 16, 77
disembedding, 76

eating disorders (EDs)
    diagnostic classification of infancy and
        early childhood, xii
    nature of, 52–53
    See also specific topics
emotional eating, 7, 8
emotion regulation, 9, 33–34
    interactive/reciprocal regulation, 9
    Mindful Emotion Regulation –
        Approach (MER-A), 2, 16, 17, 49
    problems with eating and emotion
        regulation in preschool age, 52–54
    psychotherapeutic intervention, 54–55
    regulatory processes in the cycle of life,
        8–10
    self-regulation, 9–10, 34, 68, 77, 78
Erikson, Erik H., 72
evacuation, 53, 55, 56, 58, 59
    case material, 60–64
evidence-based interventions, 12, 76

family, Minuchin's definition of the, 75
family-based interventions, 74–79
    a clinical case, 79–85
family-based therapy (FBT), 74–75
    phases, 88n7
feeding disorder associated with gastro-
    intestinal tract disorder, 36, 40, 41
    diagnostic criteria, 37t
focal play-therapy (FPT) with children
    and their parents, 55, 67–68
    "getting in the game," 62–63
        clinical vignettes, 63–67
    narrative play and, 60–62
    participated consultation (PC) and, 55,
        56, 60–63, 65
        fundamental aspects of, 61, 62
    theory and technique, 55–56, 58–60
foetal programming hypothesis, 6–7
    and the first 9 months of life:, 6–7
food neophobia, 73, 74
    defined, 73
food selectivity, 51n3
    a clinical case, 79–85
    nosographic notes, 73–74
    See also selective eating
frames, 50n1
fussy eating, 73

gastrointestinal tract disorder. *See*
    feeding disorder associated with
    gastrointestinal tract disorder

here and now (of therapy), 29, 49, 54, 55,
    67, 83, 86. *See also* present moment
homeostasis, 5, 9, 35
    of the family, 75, 80, 83, 85, 86

identity vs. role confusion (psychosocial
    development), 72
industry vs. inferiority (psychosocial
    development), 72
infantile anorexia (IA), 36, 38–44
    case material, 43–44
    diagnostic criteria, 37t
    parent–child interactions and clinical
        intervention, 43–44
intergenerational transmission. *See under*
    overweight
International Obesity Task Force
    (IOTF), 21–22
intersubjectivity, 33, 34, 54

Kerns, K.A., 72
Klein, Melanie, 60, 71n3
    case of Erna, 71n3

Lausanne Trilogue Play (LTP), 40
Leckman, James F., 36
listening, 78
Loss of Control – Eating Disorder
    (LOC-ED), 23, 30

mental awareness, fullness of, 76
mentalization, 34, 76, 77, 86, 91, 93
mentalization-based treatment (MBT), 77
mentalization-based treatment for famil-
    ies (MBT-F), 76–77, 87
micro-regulation, 33
mindful eating, 77–78
    defined, 77
Mindful Emotion Regulation –
    Approach (MER-A), 2, 16, 17, 49
mindfulness, 77, 79
    defined, 77
    See also specific topics
mindfulness-based interventions, 79. *See
    also specific interventions*
mindfulness-based relationship enhance-
    ment (MBRE), 86
mindfulness-based stress reduction
    (MBSR), 86
mindfulness processes, 76
mindful-oriented approach, 86
mindful-oriented attitude, 78

mindful parenting, 78–79, 84, 86
mindful parents, 78
Minuchin, Salvador, 74–75, 83
mismatch and reparation processes, alternating of, 9
mother–child early feeding interactions, 5
mother–child relationship, 34
motivation, 33, 34, 52–54

narrative interpretation, 60
narrative play, 60, 61
narrators within the narration, 61
nutrition, the meaning of, 5–6

overweight (and obesity)
    breastfeeding and, 23
    epidemiology, 21
    intergenerational transmission of, 24
        VIPP and, 26
    during pregnancy, 22–23
overweight in childhood and adolescence, xiv, 21–24, 29–31, 31n1
    body mass index (BMI) and, 21, 22
    case material, 26–29
    causes and risk factors, 23
    prevention of, 21, 23, 24
        starts with the relationship, 24–26
    research, 23–24
overweight mothers, 23

parental state of mind in relation to eating, 7–8
parents promoting children's awareness of hunger/satiety-related internal stimuli, 78
participated consultation (PC), 56
    case material and, 65
    Dina Vallino on, 71n2
    focal play-therapy (FPT) and, 55, 56, 60–63, 65
    overview, 55
    psychoanalysis and, 55
perinatal phase, strategies to prevent disorders during, 24
perseverant eaters, defined, 73
personification (in the play of children), 60, 71n3
picky eating, 38, 73
    defining, 73
Pine, Daniel S., 36
post-traumatic eating disorder (PTED), 38, 41–43, 47–49. See also trauma

post-traumatic feeding disorder (PTFD), 36. See also feeding disorder associated with gastrointestinal tract disorder
power. See cases: Sara and Matteo
pre-adolescence, 74
    boundaries and, 72–73
    defining, 72
pregnancy, women's weight before and during, 22–23
preschoolers. See under emotion regulation
present moment, 77
    focusing on the, 16, 29, 30, 77, 83, 86
    mindfulness and the, 16, 77, 78, 86, 89n10
    non-judgmental attitude, acceptance, and the, 2, 16, 77, 78, 86
    See also here and now
primary activity, 33
protest behaviours/protest symptoms, 53–54, 59
    case material, 28–29, 65, 81
    See also psychosomatic protest
proto-conversational readiness, 33
psychoanalysis, child, 55, 60, 71n2
psychoanalytic theory, xv, 54
psychosocial development, Erikson's stages of, 72
psychosomatic protest
    eating disorders as symptoms of, 52, 55
    See also protest behaviours/protest symptoms

reflective function of parents, 34
regulatory practices. See emotion regulation
relational selectivity, 82, 85
reparation and mismatch processes, alternating of, 9
reverie (Bion), 60

scaffolding, 34, 50n1
selective eating, 51n3
    defined, 73
    treatment, 13
    See also food selectivity
Self, 52–53
self-regulation, 9–10, 34, 68, 77, 78.
    See also emotion regulation
Selvini Palazzoli, Mara, 74–75
sensory food aversions, 36, 51n3
    diagnostic criteria, 37t

sensory food refusal, 73
separation anxiety, 41, 47–49
Solter, A., 14
structural model (family therapy), 75.
     See also Minuchin, Salvador
subjective experience, 76
     symmetrical escalation, 79

trauma, 8, 14, 37t. *See also* post-
     traumatic eating disorder
traumatic feeding experiences, 42

Vallino, Dina, 53–55, 59, 60, 71n2
video feedback, 43, 45–49
     case material, 26, 28
     use of video feedback at home,
         24–26

video-feedback intervention to
     promote positive parenting (VIPP),
     25–26

Winnicott, Donald W., 14